Debbie Indyk, PhD
Editor

The Geometry of Care: Linking Resources, Research, and Community to Reduce Degrees of Separation Between HIV Treatment and Prevention

The Geometry of Care: Linking Resources, Research, and Community to Reduce Degrees of Separation Between HIV Treatment and Prevention has been co-published simultaneously as *Social Work in Health Care*, Volume 42, Numbers 3/4 2005.

Pre-publication REVIEWS, COMMENTARIES, EVALUATIONS . . .

"**P**ROVIDES READERS WITH NEW INSIGHTS into the value of interdisciplinary collaboration to control HIV, the benefits of multilevel and ecological models for analyzing the dynamics of the epidemic, and the importance of acknowledging the multiple perspectives that different stakeholders bring to HIV care and prevention. The chapters on developing information systems and organizational infrastructures for linked prevention and treatment, and on the importance of considering the range of factors that affect adherence to medical regimens are especially useful. Finally, as low-income urban communities confront other complex epidemics such as diabetes, asthma, and depression, this book's analysis of the lessons learned from our response to HIV might provide a useful guide to research and practice."

Nicholas Freudenberg, DrPH
Distinguished Professor
Program in Urban Public Health
Hunter College
City University of New York

More Pre-publication
REVIEWS, COMMENTARIES, EVALUATIONS . . .

"This book OFFERS VERY USEFUL TOOLS based on the links between research and intervention pedagogy. It expresses careful considerations of the various steps and issues to be aware of in developing bridges to care. The authors demonstrate the need for changing the locus of expertise to optimally build the configuration of care. They also discuss best practices in integrating the expertise of all of the actors at different levels of the health care system."

Diana Rossi, DSW
Research Coordinator
Intercambios Asociación Civil
Buenos Aires, Argentina

"Dr. Indyk, a very well known and respected authority in the HIV/AIDS arena, has brought together strong evidence supporting the need for networking, coordination, and joint venturing to help us move forward in prevention and care. In this book geometry, usually a difficult subject for high-school students, is used as an exciting tool to open readers' minds toward building a productive partnership against this epidemic."

Pedro Cahn, MD, PhD
President-Elect
International AIDS Society
Chief, Infectious Diseases
Hospital Juan A. Fernandez
Director
Fundacion Huesped
Assistant Professor
Buenos Aires University
Medical School

The Haworth Press, Inc.

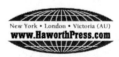

New York • London • Victoria (AU)
www.HaworthPress.com

The Geometry of Care: Linking Resources, Research, and Community to Reduce Degrees of Separation Between HIV Treatment and Prevention

The Geometry of Care: Linking Resources, Research, and Community to Reduce Degrees of Separation Between HIV Treatment and Prevention has been co-published simultaneously as *Social Work in Health Care*, Volume 42, Numbers 3/4 2006.

Monographic Separates from *Social Work in Health Care*™

For additional information on these and other Haworth Press titles, including descriptions, tables of contents, reviews, and prices, use the QuickSearch catalog at http://www.HaworthPress.com.

The Geometry of Care: Linking Resources, Research, and Community to Reduce Degrees of Separation Between HIV Treatment and Prevention, edited by Debbie Indyk, PhD (Vol. 42 3/4, 2006). *An examination of ways to link bottom-up and top-down activities to further care, services, resources, training, theory, and policy analysis for AIDS treatment and prevention.*

Bibliometrics in Social Work, edited by Gary Holden, DSW, Gary Rosenberg, PhD, and Kathleen Barker, PhD (Vol. 41, No. 3/4, 2005). *An overview of the pros and cons of using bibliometrics in social work research.*

Social Work Visions from Around the Globe: Citizens, Methods, and Approaches, edited by Anna Metteri, MSoc et al. (Vol. 39, No. 1/2 and 3/4, 2004). *"VALUABLE to practitioners in health and mental health. . . . Shows in a practical way how citizenship can be an inclusive practice related to social justice, rather than a way of excluding people from opportunities and resources in our societies." (Heather D' Cruz, PhD, MSW, Senior Lecturer in Social Work,, School of Health and Social Development, Faculty of Health and Behavioral Sciences, Deakin University, Geelong, Victoria, Australia)*

Social Work Health and Mental Health: Practice, Research and Programs, edited by Alun C. Jackson, PhD, and Steven P. Segal, PhD (Vol. 34, No. 1/2 and 3/4, 2001, and Vol. 35, No. 1/2, 2002). *Explores international perspectives on social work practice in health and mental health.*

Clinical Data-Mining in Practice-Based Research: Social Work in Hospital Settings, edited by Irwin Epstein, PhD, and Susan Blumenfield, DSW, (Vol. 33, No. 3/4, 2001). *"Challenging and illuminating. . . . This remarkable collection of exemplary studies provides inspiration and support to social workers. This book will be valuable not only as a guide to practitioners, but also is an important addition to the teaching materials for courses in social work in health care and in social research methodology." (Kay V. Davidson, DSW, Dean and Professor, University of Connecticut School of Social Work, West Hartford)*

Behavioral and Social Sciences in 21st Century Health Care: Contributions and Opportunities, edited by Gary Rosenberg, PhD, and Andrew Weissman, PhD (Vol. 33, No. 1, 2001). *"Stimulating and provocative. . . . The range of topics covered makes this book an ideal reader for health care practice courses with a combined health/mental health focus." (Goldie Kadushin, PhD, Associate Professor, School of Social Welfare, University of Wisconsin-Milwaukee)*

Seventh Doris Siegel Memorial Colloquium: Behavioral Health Care Practice in the 21st Century, edited by Gary Rosenberg, PhD, and Andrew Weissman, PhD (Vol. 31, No. 2, 2000). *"A valuable group of research studies examining important and pertinent issues. . . . Offers a fresh perspective on critical problems encountered by health care institutions, providers, patients, and families. Excellent." (Mildred D. Mailick, DSW, Professor Emerita, Hunter College School of Social Work, City University of New York)*

Social Work in Mental Health: Trends and Issues, edited by Uri Aviram (Vol. 25, No. 3, 1997). *"Suggests ways to maintain social work values in a time that emphasizes cost containment and legal requirements that may result in practices and policies that are antithetical to the profession." (Phyllis Solomon, PhD, Professor, School of Social Work, University of Pennsylvania)*

International Perspectives on Social Work in Health Care: Past, Present and Future, edited by Gail K. Auslander, DSW (Vol. 25, No. 1/2, 1997). *"The authors explore the need for new theoretical and practice models, in addition to developments in health and social work research and administration." (Council on Social Work and Education)*

Fundamentals of Perinatal Social Work: A Guide for Clinical Practice with Women, Infants, and Families, edited by Regina Furlong Lind, MSW, LCSW, and Debra Honig Bachman, MSW,

LCSW (Vol. 24, No. 3/4, 1997). *"A knowledge summation of the essence of perinatal social work that is long overdue. It is a must for any beginning perinatal social worker to own one!"* (Charlotte Collins Bursi, MSSW, Perinatal Social Worker, University of Tennessee Newborn Center; Founding President, National Association of Perinatal Social Workers)

Professional Social Work Education and Health Care: Challenges for the Future, edited by Mildred D. Mailick, DSW, and Phyllis Caroff, DSW (Vol. 24, No. 1/2, 1996). *Responds to critical concerns about the educational preparation of social workers within the rapidly changing health care environment.*

Social Work in Pediatrics, edited by Ruth B. Smith, PhD, MSW, and Helen G. Clinton, MSW (Vol. 21, No. 1, 1995). *"It presents models of service delivery and clinical practice that offer responses to the challenges of today's health care system." (Journal of Social Work Education)*

Social Work Leadership in Healthcare: Directors' Perspectives, edited by Gary Rosenberg, PhD, and Andrew Weissman, DSW (Vol. 20, No. 4, 1995). *Social work managers describe their work and work environment, detailing what qualities and traits are needed to be effective and successful now and in the future.*

Social Work in Ambulatory Care: New Implications for Health and Social Services, edited by Gary Rosenberg, PhD, and Andrew Weissman, DSW (Vol. 20, No. 1, 1994). *"A most timely book dealing with issues related to the current shift in health care delivery to ambulatory care and social work's need to position itself in this health care arena." (Barbara Berkman, DSW, Director of Research and Quality Assessment, Massachusetts General Hospital; Associate Director, Harvard Upper New England Geriatric Education Center, Harvard Medical School)*

Women's Health and Social Work: Feminist Perspectives, edited by Miriam Meltzer Olson, DSW (Vol. 19, No. 3/4, 1994). *"[Chapters] explore how social workers can better understand and address women's health, including such conditions as breast cancer, menopause, and depression. They also discuss health care centers and African-American women and AIDS." (Reference & Research Book News)*

The Changing Context of Social Health Care: Its Implications for Providers and Consumers, edited by Helen Rehr, DSW, and Gary Rosenberg, PhD (Vol. 15, No. 4, 1991). *"Required reading for every student and practitioner with a vision of improving our health care delivery system." (Candyce S. Berger, PhD, MSW, Director of Social Work, University of Washington Medical Center; Associate Professor, School of Social Work, University of Washington)*

Social Workers in Health Care Management: The Move to Leadership, edited by Gary Rosenberg, PhD, and Sylvia S. Clarke, MSc, ACSW (Vol. 12, No. 3, 1988). *"Social workers interested in hospital social work management and the potential for advancement within the health care field will find the book interesting and challenging as well as helpful." (Social Thought)*

Social Work and Genetics: A Guide to Practice, edited by Sylvia Schild, DSW, and Rita Beck Black, DSW (Supp #1, 1984). *"Precisely defines the responsibilities of social work in the expanding field of medical genetics and presents a clear, comprehensive overview of basic genetic principles and issues." (Health and Social Work)*

Advancing Social Work Practice in the Health Care Field: Emerging Issues and New Perspectives, edited by Gary Rosenberg, PhD, and Helen Rehr, DSW (Vol. 8, No. 3, 1983). *"Excellent articles, useful bibliographies, and additional reading lists." (Australian Social Work)*

Published by

The Haworth Press Inc., 10 Alice Street, Binghamton, NY 13904-1580 USA

The Geometry of Care: Linking Resources, Research, and Community to Reduce Degrees of Separation Between HIV Treatment and Prevention has been co-published simultaneously as *Social Work in Health Care,* Volume 42, Numbers 3/4 2006.

The development, preparation, and publication of this work has been undertaken with great care. However, the publisher, employees, editors, and agents of The Haworth Press and all imprints of The Haworth Press, Inc., including The Haworth Medical Press® and Pharmaceutical Products Press®, are not responsible for any errors contained herein or for consequences that may ensue from use of materials or information contained in this work. With regard to case studies, identities and circumstances of individuals discussed herein have been changed to protect confidentiality. Any resemblance to actual persons, living or dead, is entirely coincidental.

The Haworth Press is committed to the dissemination of ideas and information according to the highest standards of intellectual freedom and the free exchange of ideas. Statements made and opinions expressed in this publication do not necessarily reflect the views of the Publisher, Directors, management, or staff of The Haworth Press, Inc., or an endorsement by them.

Cover design by Jennifer Gaska

Library of Congress Cataloging-in-Publication Data

The geometry of care: linking resources, research, and community to reduce degrees of separation between HIV treatment and prevention/ Debbie Indyk, PhD.
     p. cm.
     "has been co-published simultaneously as Social work in health care, volume 42, numbers 3/4 2006"
     Includes bibliographical references and index.
     ISBN 13: 978-0-7890-3211-9 (hard cover : alk. paper)
     ISBN 10: 0-7890-3211-2 (hard cover : alk. paper)
     ISBN 13: 978-0-7890-3212-6 (soft cover : alk paper)
     ISBN 10: 0-7890-3212-0 (soft cover : alk. paper)
     1. DNLM: HIV infections–Treatment. 2. Community health services. I. Indyk, Debbie. II. Social work in health care.
     1. HIV Infections–prevention & control. 2. Community Health Services. Health Promotion. 4. Primary Prevention. W1 SO 135P v. 42 no. 3/4 2006 / WC 503.6 G345 2006]
RC607.A26G46 2005
362.196'9792–dc22
          2005031505

The Geometry of Care:
Linking Resources,
Research, and Community
to Reduce Degrees
of Separation
Between HIV Treatment
and Prevention

Debbie Indyk, PhD
Editor
Gary Rosenberg, PhD
Andrew Weissman, PhD
Series Editors

The Geometry of Care: Linking Resources, Research, and Community to Reduce Degrees of Separation Between HIV Treatment and Prevention has been co-published simultaneously as *Social Work in Health Care*, Volume 42, Numbers 3/4 2006.

The Haworth Press, Inc.

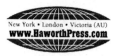

New York • London • Victoria (AU)
www.HaworthPress.com

Indexing, Abstracting & Website/Internet Coverage

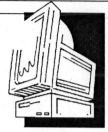

This section provides you with a list of major indexing & abstracting services and other tools for bibliographic access. That is to say, each service began covering this periodical during the year noted in the right column. Most Websites which are listed below have indicated that they will either post, disseminate, compile, archive, cite or alert their own Website users with research-based content from this work. (This list is as current as the copyright date of this publication.)

Abstracting, Website/Indexing Coverage . . . . Year When Coverage Began

- *Abstracts in Social Gerontology: Current Literature on Aging* **1989**
- *Academic Abstracts/CD-ROM* **1995**
- *Academic Search Elite (EBSCO)* **2001**
- *Academic Search Premier (EBSCO)*
  <http://www.epnet.com/academic/acasearchprem.asp> **1994**
- *AgeLine Database <http://research.aarp.org/ageline>* **2000**
- *Applied Social Sciences Index & Abstracts (ASSIA) (Online: ASSI via DataStar) (CDRom: ASSIA Plus)*
  <http://www.csa.com> **1987**
- *Behavioral Medicine Abstracts (Annals of Behavioral Medicine)* **1983**
- *Behavioral Medicine Abstracts (Pain Evaluation and Treatment Institute)* **1997**
- *Business Source Corporate: coverage of nearly 3,350 quality magazines and journals; designed to meet the diverse information needs of corporation; EBSCO Publishing <http://www.epnet.com/corporate/bsourcecorp.asp>* . . **1994**
- *CareData: the database supporting social care management and pratice <http://www.elsc.org.uk/caredata/caredata.htm>* **1975**
- *CINAHL (Cumulative Index to Nursing & Allied Health Literature), in print, EBSCO, and SilverPlatter, DataStar, and PaperChase. (Support materials include Subject Heading List, Database Search Guide, and instructional video)*
  <http://www.cinahl.com> **1981**

(continued)

(continued)

(continued)

Special Bibliographic Notes related to special journal issues (separates) and indexing/abstracting:

- indexing/abstracting services in this list will also cover material in any "separate" that is co-published simultaneously with Haworth's special thematic journal issue or DocuSerial. Indexing/abstracting usually covers material at the article/chapter level.
- monographic co-editions are intended for either non-subscribers or libraries which intend to purchase a second copy for their circulating collections.
- monographic co-editions are reported to all jobbers/wholesalers/approval plans. The source journal is listed as the "series" to assist the prevention of duplicate purchasing in the same manner utilized for books-in-series.
- to facilitate user/access services all indexing/abstracting services are encouraged to utilize the co-indexing entry note indicated at the bottom of the first page of each article/chapter/contribution.
- this is intended to assist a library user of any reference tool (whether print, electronic, online, or CD-ROM) to locate the monographic version if the library has purchased this version but not a subscription to the source journal.
- individual articles/chapters in any Haworth publication are also available through the Haworth Document Delivery Service (HDDS).

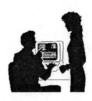

The Geometry of Care: Linking Resources, Research, and Community to Reduce Degrees of Separation Between HIV Treatment and Prevention

CONTENTS

ABOUT THE EDITOR

Debbie Indyk, PhD, MS, is Associate Professor in the Department of Community and Preventive Medicine at the Mount Sinai School of Medicine and serves simultaneously as Director of Education and Prevention of the Mount Sinai Medical Center (MSMC) AIDS Center. Dr. Indyk trained in public health, sociology and information science at Columbia University. Dr. Indyk is Principal Investigator of the Mount Sinai/Argentina Fogarty AITRP and of Health Bridge, an innovative clinical outreach program designed to find and engage HIV infected individuals who are not in care. She was a lecturer at Columbia University Mailman School of Public Health where she has taught a course in Community Health Development which provides a self-exemplifying case study of "how to link bottom-up, top-down" activities to advance-services, resources, training and policy analysis. She mentors many students in field-placed training including street outreach, needle exchange programs and home-visiting programs.

Her accomplishment has been to break new ground in the theoretical explanation of the requisites for AIDS knowledge production and integration. Dr. Indyk has convincingly demonstrated that actors at no single level or site–or type of site–command expertise sufficient to address the full range of problems on the prevention-detection-treatment-cure continuum: Each has his (or her) own expertise. Her special contribution has been to add to the understanding of organizational structures that are required to effectively respond to new diseases and the medical advances that they spawn. Her experience with grassroots organizations and their insights, as well as the theoretical models resulting from these collaborations, enable her to offer the same "bottom-up and top-down" blueprint, evolved through treatment programs, prevention initiatives and collaboration with researchers. At the same time, she has been able to serve both traditional and unique educational roles.

Her work supports the development of community-based sites as knowledge producers. Each site provides a setting in which to develop and validate interventions for administration, grassroots providers, and clients. Thus, a family health service is identified as a site to reach pregnant women; a Union Health Center is a site for reaching those at risk for TB; and a needle exchange program affords access to those with/at risk for HIV and TB. The sustained relationship with each agency permits the exchange, assessment, and integration of emerging early intervention and prevention information. This helps in customizing appropriate interventions, in deciding how best to secure and deliver necessary resources, and in evaluating program efficacy. Often, evaluation involves creation of data management capacity to track who is served, how they are served, and where these clients go next in the system. Such elements also permit generation and testing of hypotheses. Through this service driven program development and evaluation work, Dr. Indyk has successfully created multi-millions of infrastructure support dollars for community-based organizations which she continues to support after funding to collaborate in the development, implementation and evaluation of this model.

Acknowledgments

I have been extremely fortunate to work with many individuals who have made the work presented in this issue possible. Renate Belville, was my mentor and the collaborator who helped to direct my work outward in the community where she and Jane Moss had worked so effectively to support capacity building efforts in East Harlem. Little Sisters of the Assumption Family Health Service (LSA), Dominican Sisters Family Health Service (DSFHS), Health Bridge, the East Harlem HIV Care Network and Mount Sinai's AIDS Center provided strategic sites through which to develop this model.

At various times two former graduate research associates, Drs. David Rier and Sarit Golub, have played instrumental roles in the elaboration of this work.

My sincere appreciation is extended to Peggy Sweeney, administrator of Dominican Sisters with whom I have had the privilege to work over the past 14 years to support the development of a dynamic community-based model for providing access to a continuum of prevention and treatment services which is highly responsive to community, staff and client needs.

The most highly developed example of this model, Health Bridge, was initially conceived and developed jointly with Karyn London and implemented and sustained by other members of the Health Bridge team: Ann Boyer, Alicene Pilgrim, Melisha Owens and Donnie White. They have created and sustained webs of linkages to connect-the-dots between hard-to-reach clients and services they need and are willing, able and ready to obtain.

Currently, Dr. Alejandra Gurtman, Dr. Henry Sacks, Gizelle Kiperman and George Carter and collaborators in Argentina and India are ap-

[Haworth co-indexing entry note]: "Acknowledgments." Co-published simultaneously in *Social Work in Health Care* (The Haworth Press, Inc.) Vol. 42, No. 3/4, 2006, pp. xxxi-xxxii; and: *The Geometry of Care: Linking Resources, Research, and Community to Reduce Degrees of Separation Between HIV Treatment and Prevention* (ed: Debbie Indyk) The Haworth Press, Inc., 2006, pp. xvii-xviii. Single or multiple copies of this article are available for a fee from The Haworth Document Delivery Service [1-800-HAWORTH, 9:00 a.m. - 5:00 p.m. (EST). E-mail address: docdelivery@haworthpress.com].

doi:10.1300/J010v42n03

plying and extending this top-down bottom-up framework to support capacity building efforts in Argentina and India. Much of this work has been made possible through an NIH Fogarty AIDS International Training and Research program which has supported the training of almost 50 Argentinean practitioners to integrate research into practice in order to effect change at the micro and macro levels. Their work is being documented and presented through other forums.

Drs. Helen Rehr and Gary Rosenberg have patiently provided encouragement and support. This issue would not have been executed without them.

Finally, my lifelong collaborator and spouse, Dr. Len Indyk, has provided direction and support in the creation of information systems crafted to meet and be responsive to the developmental needs of the agencies as required by this model. He serves as my greatest mentor, sounding board and critic.

Debbie Indyk, PhD

Overview of Issue

Debbie Indyk

In this volume we present a self-exemplifying case study of how to link bottom-up and top down activities to advance care, services, resources, training, theory, and policy analysis. Over the past seventeen years, through work with community-based organizations both locally and internationally, I and my collaborators have focused on developing and sustaining the structures and processes necessary to harness, assess and effectively disseminate new knowledge so that it can be incorporated into practice. This system-building and evaluation work draws on behavioral and organizational theory to support sustained development and evaluation with community-based organizations (CBOs) serving populations at high risk for TB and HIV/AIDS. As Director of Education and Prevention for the Mount Sinai AIDS Center and Associate Professor in the Department of Community and Preventive Medicine, I have been positioned to straddle both medical center and community, prevention and treatment and theory and practice.

During the early phases of the AIDS epidemic, working closely with David Rier, we realized that "AIDS knowledge" was produced by a wide range of actors, including not only scientists and clinicians, but also front-line workers and consumers. We argued that networks which distribute new knowledge must extend past community hospitals and physicians, to those "in the trenches," who are often the true experts in their specific fields. These include: social workers, drug counselors, sex educators, community-outreach workers, the staffs of needle-exchange programs, food pantries and soup kitchens, and consumers, whose locus

---

[Haworth co-indexing entry note]: "Overview of Issue." Indyk, Debbie. Co-published simultaneously in *Social Work in Health Care* (The Haworth Press, Inc.) Vol. 42, No. 3/4, 2006, pp. 1-6; and: *The Geometry of Care: Linking Resources, Research, and Community to Reduce Degrees of Separation Between HIV Treatment and Prevention* (ed: Debbie Indyk) The Haworth Press, Inc., 2006, pp. 1-6. Single or multiple copies of this article are available for a fee from The Haworth Document Delivery Service [1-800-HAWORTH, 9:00 a.m. - 5:00 p.m. (EST). E-mail address: docdelivery@haworthpress.com].

Available online at http://www.haworthpress.com/web/SWHC
doi:10.1300/J010v42n03_01

affords them unique insights and knowledge which *complements* that produced by others. As the epidemic matured, the burden of illness-management and transmission-prevention shifted to the infected individual. The challenge of identifying, engaging and retaining hard-to-reach individuals in care has become increasingly critical to the future face of the epidemic.

The work in this special volume rests on several related insights. First, that changing the *focus* of a problem means changing the *locus* of the expertise relevant to address it. Thus, for example, while the ultimate cure for AIDS may come from basic scientists, community-based providers–with their access to, trust commanded among, and familiarity with at-risk populations–are often the experts in designing realistic prevention interventions. Second is the corollary point that each aspect, each phase of a problem, has its own set of experts. This leads to the third, and central insight, that addressing complex sociomedical problems such as TB or AIDS requires linkage between these disparate types of providers and sites, and mechanisms by which all types of providers–and patients–can exchange their unique observations and harness their respective expertise in prevention, education, research, and service. A final major insight flowing from this work is the overwhelming importance of cultivating the proper site for each given function–prevention, education, research and service. Shifting the locus of care along the continuum of prevention and treatment requires a major shift in the 'geometry of care.'

The framework for this volume–The Geometry of Care: Linking Resources, Research and Community to Reduce Degrees of Separation between HIV Treatment and Prevention–stresses the extent to which both treatment and prevention are critical elements in the continuum of care, and must be integrated and linked. *The Supplement is divided into two parts. Part I focuses on System- and Program-Level Geometry and part II on Patient and Provider Level Geometry.*

The Rationale of Inter-Organizational Linkages (Rier and Indyk) provides the theoretic framework for this new geometry: broadening the vanguard of care to include community and patients, interdependence between community and medical center, and a shift from a top-down approach to knowledge production and dissemination to a multi-frontal approach requiring sustained intra- and inter-organizational webs. These support harnessing assessment, dissemination and integration of new advances along the continuum of risk and prevention.

The approach fosters the bottom-up development of a web of linkages among providers, systems and settings. Communication with the network of highly skilled generalists and specialists within the hospital framework allows for intensive client care at all levels of client readiness and medical need. In *Wiring the HIV/AIDS System: Building Infrastructure to Link People, Sites, and Networks* (Indyk and Rier), the authors provide examples of this linkage and infrastructure building at a family health service, a medical center-based AIDS center, and a home-based ambulatory care program which provides outreach, engagement and retention in clinical care to a critical mass of individuals with HIV/AIDS living in Single Room Occupancy Hotels who are not in care.

Indyk and Indyk, in *Collecting Data Along the Continuum of Prevention and Care: A Continuous Quality Improvement Approach*, describe how the sustained relationship with each setting and site permitted the exchange, assessment, and integration of emerging early intervention and prevention information. This relationship helped in customizing appropriate interventions, in deciding how best to secure and deliver necessary resources, and in evaluating program efficacy. Often, evaluation involved creation of data management capacity to help agencies track those they are serving, understand how clients are being served, and where these clients go next in the system. With the shifting vanguard, data analysis is not only required by academics, but also by CBOs doing cutting edge work in the community.

Many of the individuals in need of HIV care also require substance abuse treatment services and re-entry support after incarceration. Prevention and treatment must be integrated, not only to support HIV care, but also to support care for individuals confronting multiple co-morbidities (such as addictions) and challenges. In *A Community-Based Organization's Integration of HIV and Substance Abuse Treatment Services for Ex-Offenders,* Strauss describes how an agency, VIP Community Services, has moved to *integrate* services for this difficult and needy population, requiring the adoption of many aspects of the approach outlined in by Rier and Indyk.

In *Culture, Community Networks, and HIV/AIDS Outreach Opportunities in a South Indian Siddha Organization,* Baban and colleagues, apply this model on an international level. This article was developed as part of an assessment and feasibility study to evaluate the efficacy of an indigenous (Siddha) medication that is used by practitioners to treat HIV. Redefining the vanguard can mean forging linkages between Western and traditional medicine. However, differences between core Siddha traditional beliefs and Western prevention and treatment beliefs and practices are so fundamental that these 'degrees of separation' must be reduced substantially before many of these linkages can be established and strengthened to maximize each region's ability to reach and engage individuals in prevention and treatment.

In the final article in Part I, in *Requisites, Benefits, and Challenges of Sustainable HIV/AIDS System-Building: Where Theory Meets Practice*, Indyk and Rier offer organizational requisites to conducting this work, so that others can adapt and apply the linkage approach to manage HIV/AIDS or other problems. We explain how theory and practice have driven one another in this work.

Part II focuses on *Patient-Level Geometry: Adherence and Uncertainty–The Challenge of Practicing Change While Changing Practice*. Supporting adherence to a more positive lifestyle for individuals living with multiple layers of needs also necessitates meeting them "where they are." Prevention strategies must be tailored to meet people wherever they are located on three continuums, including: the at-risk infected continuum, the life cycle continuum, and the degree of awareness continuum regarding the problem and the need for prevention and risk reduction. Prevention is a process, is incremental, and requires changing practice and practicing change on the parts of client, providers, and settings. This multi-dimensional and multi-stage framework allows for the simultaneous and discrete assessment of intervention efficacy at various settings and various stages of health and disease.

In *The Shifting Locus of Risk-Reduction: The Critical Role of HIV Infected Individuals, Indyk and Golub argue that the convergence of prevention and treatment shifts the locus of care to the HIV-positive individual, who must simultaneously manage primary, secondary and tertiary risk-reduction. This further supports the need for a new geometry of care.*

Rier and Indyk in *Flexible Rigidity: Supporting HIV Treatment Adherence in a Rapidly-Changing Treatment Environment*, provide a rationale for a new adherence paradigm based on 5 years of experience with changing regimens, technologies and emerging knowledge. Extension of the model to the patient-level requires a flexible approach to treatment and an inter-organizational approach to supporting and sustaining patient-provider interaction.

Boyer and Indyk argue in *Shaping Garments of Care: Tools for Maximizing Adherence Potential* that successful adherence can only be accomplished by rethinking what constitutes 'care,' and 'tailoring' that care to the individual. In this context, adherence requires the interweaving of three sets of needs: (1) needs perceived by the client, (2) client needs as observed by an objective recorder and assessed for impact on the client's ability and willingness to be adherent, and (3) medical needs identified by an impartial clinician. The work has led to the creation of a Cluster of Tools (HIVCOT) which is offered to support individual adjustments to the design of care such that it closely fits the abilities of the client and maximizes the potential for adherence.

Individualized care design means understanding the demands of care, and listening to what patients mean by 'adherence.' Golub and colleagues in *Reframing HIV Adherence as Part of the Experience of Illness* suggest an alternative frame for understanding barriers to adherence which focuses on: (1) the meaning that adherence/pill-taking behavior has for individuals experiencing chronic illness; and (2) the impact that this behavior has on their identity.

The complexity of the issues affecting adherence to a pediatric HIV medical regimen can overwhelm both the practitioner and the patient. By utilizing a developmental framework and emphasizing the critical importance of the relationship among provider, patient and family. In *Pediatric HIV Adherence: An Ever-Evolving Challenge,* Childs and Cincotta present HIV as a family disease, and the geometry of care as a family issue.

Apollo and colleagues in *Patient-Provider Relationships,* HIV and Adherence: Requisites for a Partnership focus on yet another aspect of this geometry of care. Patient cooperation alone, long viewed as both necessary and sufficient to support adherent behavior, is wholly inadequate, in this rapidly changing environment. With the locus of care management shifting along the continuum of risk and disease, a partnership must be forged between the patient and his primary care provider to help the patient be proactively involved in both health maintenance and disease management.

Golub and Indyk demonstrate that the shifting locus of care logically leads to a redefinition of the partner notification process, so as to include *HIV Infected Individuals as Partners in Prevention.* People living with HIV disease, who are instrumentally involved in their care, are clearly strategically positioned to prevent both transmission and acquisition of the virus. Prevention is a *process*, not an outcome. An effective geometry of care simultaneously supports public health and individual needs.

Management of HIV can be prescribed by medical providers, but can only be accomplished through client "adherence" to these recommendations. Individuals *already* infected need to be supported in their acceptance and management of these complex issues; they may need support with recovery, family, daily activities, finance, and health as well as to develop and maintain safer behaviors. Many of these individuals are simultaneously dealing other serious conditions such as addiction, Hepatitis and other chronic illnesses. Many individuals are vulnerable because of post traumatic stress disorder, domestic violence, substance use, HIV, mental illness and other stressors. For those whose risk has been stabilized, relapse prevention is needed. For those at high-risk of relapse (from engagement in care, medication regimen and sexual risk behavior) additional intensive "prevention" treatments are needed to support maintenance of targeted behavior. The new geometry of care links resources, research and community to fully integrate HIV prevention and treatment and help infected individuals live longer and healthier lives.

Finally, in *The STARK Study: A Cross-Sectional Study of Adherence to Short-Term Drug Regimens in Urban Kenya*, the authors describe an adherence study conducted in a resource poor neighborhood in Nairobi which demonstrated that a community-based clinic with committed healthcare workers in Kenya can empower an economically disadvantaged population to be adherent. This free clinic model holds much promise in the future for bridging communities to HIV prevention and treatment.

PART I

SYSTEM-
AND PROGRAM-LEVEL
GEOMETRY

The Rationale of Interorganizational Linkages to Connect Multiple Sites of Expertise, Knowledge Production, and Knowledge Transfer: An Example from HIV/AIDS Services for the Inner City

David A. Rier, PhD
Debbie Indyk, PhD

David A. Rier, PhD, is affiliated with the Department of Sociology and Anthropology, Bar-Ilan University, Ramat-Gan, Israel. Debbie Indyk is affiliated with the Department of Community and Preventive Medicine, Mount Sinai School of Medicine, New York, NY.

Address correspondence to: Debbie Indyk, PhD, Department of Community and Preventive Medicine, Box 1045, Mount Sinai School of Medicine, One Gustave Levy Place, New York, NY 10029 (E-mail: debbie_indyk@mssm.edu).

The authors are indebted to Professors Renate Belville, Steven Epstein, Mary Fennell, Ann Flood, Bruce V. Lewenstein, and Michael Harrison for their valuable suggestions, and to Katie Courtice and Wendy J. Harris for technical assistance.

Much earlier versions of portions of this paper were presented to the American Sociological Association, 88th Annual Meeting, August 13-17, 1993, Miami Beach, FL, and to the American Public Health Association, 122nd Annual Meeting, Washington, DC, Oct. 30-Nov. 3, 1994.

[Haworth co-indexing entry note]: "The Rationale of Interorganizational Linkages to Connect Multiple Sites of Expertise, Knowledge Production, and Knowledge Transfer: An Example from HIV/AIDS Services for the Inner City." Rier, David A., and Debbie Indyk. Co-published simultaneously in *Social Work in Health Care* (The Haworth Press, Inc.) Vol. 42, No. 3/4, 2006, pp. 9-27; and: *The Geometry of Care: Linking Resources, Research, and Community to Reduce Degrees of Separation Between HIV Treatment and Prevention* (ed: Debbie Indyk) The Haworth Press, Inc., 2006, pp. 9-27. Single or multiple copies of this article are available for a fee from The Haworth Document Delivery Service [1-800-HAWORTH, 9:00 a.m. - 5:00 p.m. (EST). E-mail address: docdelivery@haworthpress.com].

SUMMARY. This paper presents the rationale for a long-running project in which various community-based and tertiary-based providers are being linked to each other in order to understand, reach, and engage high-risk, hard-to-reach inner-city residents for prevention, treatment, and management of HIV/AIDS. Not simply a *program* to link disparate actors, the work has developed into a more fundamental *approach* through which to build and maintain the infrastructure required to generate and sustain knowledge development and integration within and between systems. This work is grounded in the recognition that each type of provider, as well as patients and clients themselves, has a particular type of expertise. All forms of expertise are necessary to fight HIV/AIDS. Different forms of expertise are necessary to diagnose, treat, prevent, and cure HIV/AIDS and its sequelae. This work suggests revisions in traditional approaches to expertise and to the content and geometry of dissemination networks, and ultimately challenges the very concepts of dissemination and the lay/scientific boundary. *[Article copies available for a fee from The Haworth Document Delivery Service: 1-800-HAWORTH. E-mail address: <docdelivery@haworthpress.com> Website: <http://www.HaworthPress.com> © 2006 by The Haworth Press, Inc. All rights reserved.]*

KEYWORDS. AIDS, organizations, dissemination, networks, sociology of science, sociology of knowledge

WHO IS WISE? HE WHO LEARNS FROM EVERY PERSON (TALMUD)

Sociomedical phenomena as complex as HIV/AIDS generally require forms of expertise and insight more varied than any one type of provider or institution can offer. The relevant experts are not found only in laboratories or lecture halls: they include street-level drug treatment workers, and are found, too, amongst clients and patients. Each party involved in HIV/AIDS occupies a specific social location affording unique insights, and enabling the production of unique knowledge that complements and supplements knowledge produced elsewhere.

This diversity of knowledge and experience suggests broader implications for an insight made long ago about scientific expertise:

> Every discipline, in fact every problem, has its own *vanguard*, the group of research scientists working practically on a given problem. This is followed by the *main body*, the official community.... The vanguard does not occupy a fixed position. It changes its quarters from day to day and even from hour to hour. (Fleck [1935] 1979:124)

The fight against AIDS is composed of numerous such core-periphery sets. Initially, the effort against HIV placed virologists as the vanguard in pursuit of a "magic bullet" with which to defeat the disease. However, as hopes for a quick cure faded, the focus turned to improved treatment/management, making infectious disease specialists the new vanguard. With the advent of combination therapy, AIDS evolved from an acute disease, treated via hospitalization, to a chronic condition managed on an out-patient basis in the community, making community-based providers the new vanguard. Each change in the *focus* of the fight against HIV requires a parallel shift in the *locus* of expertise, from the university laboratory to the medical center to the community. As the focus shifts even further toward integrating treatment and prevention, it is primary care physicians and community-based sociomedical providers–with their sustained contact with and deeper insight into their patients and clients–who are best equipped to represent the vanguard of a newly defined problem. And, especially in inner cities, neither treatment nor prevention is possible without outreach to find and engage those outside the care system. This shift toward engaging the hard to reach and/or those who may be engaged and then lost to the system demands the expertise of not only community-based providers, but also the patients/clients themselves, whose insights into their situation are crucial to designing realistic, effective interventions.

Vital though they are, then, research scientists and clinical specialists are not always at the vanguard of AIDS knowledge. Rather, expertise is distributed across multiple boundaries of function, discipline, and location. As Fleck taught, the site of relevant expertise changes with the particular question. Early signs and symptoms of disease are not likely to be observed by researchers working in a medical center. They cannot be identified without the input from a critical mass of individuals positioned to observe these signs and begin systematically to sort them out. Community-based organizations working in the trenches at the height of the crack epidemic in the late 1980s were the first to recognize and report "crack babies." In recent years, grassroots laymen and community-based activists have helped design and conduct their own clinical

AIDS trials, and laymen have become acknowledged experts in technical areas of AIDS (Epstein, 1995, 1996; Arno and Feiden, 1992; Nussbaum, 1990; Indyk and Rier, 1993).

As with knowledge and expertise, so with innovation: not sharing researchers' commitment to rigorous research methods, community providers may sometimes prove the more creative in identifying and addressing local problems (Rotheram-Borus, Rebchook, Kelly, Adams, and Neumann, 2000). Frontline knowledge production is often fueled by emergent needs identified by workers and by the indigenous resources and technology available to them on a day-to-day basis. Codified 'standards of care' are often adapted and modified to meet local realities. In this environment new knowledge is obtained, assessed, and incorporated into practice by workers. Another key feature of HIV/AIDS that contributes to the shifting of the vanguard is that clients'/patients' disparate needs are neither easily predicted nor always sequential. HIV-infected individuals often experience acute episodes requiring hospitalization and intensive medical care, but then can be sent home, where they might require anything from minimal to extensive sociomedical support services. Many individuals simultaneously need job training, substance use treatment, preventive services, and sophisticated hospital care. Family members are also affected by a patient's illness, and may even be infected themselves, requiring additional services. Even once engaged by the system, clients may fall out of care at any stage of the disease.

Combined with the realities of severe fragmentation of existing systems and resources, the shifting locus of expertise and the disparate needs of HIV-positive individuals render crucial the capacity to develop, modify, and maintain rich inter-organizational and inter-system linkages. Only through such linkages is it possible to make most effective use of providers, resources, and expertise. But even numerous such point-to-point linkages are not enough. In order to tap and distribute the expertise specific to *each* point in the system (whether medical school, community-based organization [CBO], client, etc.), inter-organizational linkages must be developed into wider networks and ultimately *webs* of linkages. In such a web, each particular site ideally constitutes a hub (node) that harnesses, assesses, consumes, and produces knowledge. Moreover, it must be supplied with the linkage infrastructure necessary to modify and sustain this flow in an environment of fluid demands and opportunities.

Since 1989, the second author has been constructing and implementing such a system from the ground up. This has entailed building inter-organizational linkages and infrastructure to prevent, manage, and

treat HIV/AIDS via needs assessment, program development and implementation, and evaluation. Her work began with the recognition that
such linkages were necessary to give the high-risk, hard-to-reach residents of such New York City neighborhoods as East Harlem and the
South Bronx access both to community-based organizations and to a
major medical center.

Initially, Mount Sinai Medical Center was conceived as the vanguard–the hub through which community providers were linked with
the necessary resources (technical, clinical, educational) to better reach
and serve their population. Gradually, however, it became clear that the
job was not merely to link disadvantaged communities to sociomedical
services. Nor was it merely to enable top-down dissemination of resources and insights from credentialed experts to the front-line, grassroots providers serving inner-city communities. Instead, this early
vision eventually evolved into efforts to create the web described
above–multiple nodes that each can shift its role from vanguard to
main-body, depending on the nature of the problem (and proposed solutions). In practice, much of the work has been the development of infrastructure (such as forums, committees, and collaborative agreements) to
generate and sustain the diverse linkages comprising this web.

Below, we use this work to inform a new approach through which to
build and maintain infrastructure designed to generate and sustain
knowledge development and integration within and between systems.
Other articles in this volume present case-studies from our own and others' work demonstrating how the approach may be applied. This new
approach uses the diversity of expertise and shifting vanguard as the rationale for forging linkages within and between systems and redefining
the geometry of dissemination networks. In fact, we will raise questions
about the validity of the concept of dissemination, itself, and about the
border between credentialed scientists and non-scientists in the new
geometry of care.

THE PROBLEMS:
TROUBLED POPULATION, COMPLEX DISEASE,
FRAGMENTARY RESPONSE

Residents of American inner-city communities often fall through the
cracks of a badly fragmented health care system. Such residents frequently interact only sporadically, if at all, with the medical system.
Certainly there is grinding poverty, with its implications for housing,

nutrition, and other basic resources. Often, there are also: language barriers; histories of past and current illicit substance abuse; problems of undocumented immigration; histories of emotional and mental problems; and unstable, abusive domestic arrangements. Combined with financial and cultural barriers, there are also numerous spatial, temporal, and bureaucratic obstacles (such as often-changing, conflicting eligibility requirements) arising from the typically hodgepodge nature of services. These factors greatly complicate detection, engagement, and retention of such individuals in medical or social services. Prevention, early diagnosis, and management of HIV/AIDS in this population thus require sustained outreach and service coordination.

Consider the two New York City communities that have been the main foci of our activities, East Harlem (in Manhattan) and Mott Haven (in the South Bronx). New York City "continues to be the epicenter of the HIV/AIDS epidemic in the U.S." (New York City Commission on HIV/AIDS, 2005:4). Within the city, East Harlem ranks first, and Hunts Point/Mott Haven fourth, of 42 neighborhoods in the rate of AIDS mortality (New York City Department of Health and Mental Hygiene, 2005a). These two neighborhoods have rates of AIDS- and drug-related deaths and hospitalizations 2.5-3.5 times the city average (New York City Department of Health and Mental Hygiene, 2005b, 2005c). City-wide, 30% of those diagnosed with HIV in the first half of 2004 were diagnosed concurrently with AIDS (New York City Department of Health and Mental Hygiene, 2005d:2). In other words, these individuals had endured the typically-long latency period without being aware they had the virus until they were actually sick with AIDS, itself. Current overall estimates are that 25% of HIV+ New Yorkers have never been tested, and hence are unaware of their status (New York City Department of Health and Mental Hygiene, 2005d:1).

Early diagnosis and intervention can both prolong life and prevent transmission of the virus. CBOs, with their familiarity with and access to the daily lives of those most at risk, are well-positioned for outreach and frontline service duties. However, CBOs frequently wrestle with problems such as severe resource constraints and staff turnover (Chillag, Bartholow, Cordeiro, Swanson et al., 2002; Kelly, Sogolow, and Neumann, 2000). Moreover, HIV/AIDS clients' needs often exceed what CBOs are normally configured to provide. After being assessed for risk, clients must be linked to sustained service and treatment regimens. Complex clinical management and treatment, typically dependent on highly specialized skills and other costly resources, normally require medical centers, organizations that are highly hierarchical and bureaucratic.

The complementary functions and scales of community-based providers (who, in the inner city, often fulfill monitoring and support functions normally performed, elsewhere, by family members) and the medical center evoke Tonnies' ([1887]1993) classic distinction between *gemeinschaft* (community) and *gesellschaft* (society). Tonnies used these terms to explain two phases of historical social development, involving a shift from a world based on intimate primary group ties (community) to one based on impersonal, bureaucratized rationality (society). Tonnies intended the *gemeinschaft/gesellschaft* distinction to be used as a tool for further research (Heberle, 1993). In this spirit, we adopt his concept as a tool to explain, not successive phases of development, but concurrent types of organizational roles (see also: Nisbet and Perrin, 1977; Holland, 1964; Martindale, 1960; Adler, Kwon, and Signer, 2003).

The *focus* of HIV/AIDS clients' needs often shifts between prevention, basic social services, and complex medical and mental health treatment. As such, the appropriate *locus* of support shifts between the community and medical center–and back again. These disparate functions and services, the sites and providers that offer them, and the systems that support them, are linked tenuously (at best). Though the discussion that follows focuses on the importance of linking community and tertiary resources, it is not only the medical center and the community that need to be joined to one another. At times, the gulf between various medical center units (such as those between Psychiatry, Infectious Disease, and Cardiology) with stakes in AIDS work may be larger even than that between community and medical center. Different specialties and disciplines often have vastly different approaches and interests. Sometimes these are non-overlapping, other times there may be direct competition. In either case, forging and coordinating an integrated response to HIV/AIDS is rarely simple.

Taking all the various disjunctions into account, it is not surprising that many potential patients never manage to connect with or navigate the systems involved. This is particularly frustrating today, when medicine finally offers powerful tools for holding AIDS at bay. Part of the problem lies in the medical center's size and impersonality (as well as its weak, often troubled ties with the community), which can distance and exclude both inner city clients and community providers. Moreover, medical center-based providers' perceptions of inner city life are sometimes skewed by stereotypes and naïveté. Earlier in the epidemic, for example, academic physicians did not always grasp that inner city families might rank steam heat or food stamps as higher priorities than HIV testing. Such ignorance of context can doom interventions (McLeroy, Bibeau, Steckler et al., 1988), particularly in the absence of good will between community and medical center. Whether involving HIV testing, clinical trials enrollment, prevention, or treatment, community distrust and resentment of the medical establishment run deep. Indeed, mistrust runs both ways (Gross, 1993). Conversely, rapport with clients is a particular strength of CBOs.

THE SOLUTION: BUILDING BRIDGES, AND FROM BRIDGES TO WEBS

Figure 1 frames the following discussion of our solution to these problems, and its theoretical significance.

Interorganizational linkages for diffusion of medical advances have traditionally been conceived in top-down fashion, in which academic researchers send their innovation down to community-based clinicians (Figure 1a). A key example was the National Institutes of Health (NIH) cancer dissemination network demonstration model of the 1970s, in which academic physician-researchers based in tertiary-level medical centers transmitted cancer treatment innovations to physician-practitioners located in community hospitals (Fennell and Warnecke, 1988). This work advanced thinking on dissemination by highlighting the value of interorganizational networks to this process.

Yet such a model scarcely taps the full potential of interorganizational linkages. First, since the NIH model defined community physicians as fairly passive adopters, and not as producers of information, it failed to capture these providers' insights. There was no input from the community-based physicians, to say nothing of non-physician community providers or patients. This is the traditional approach of the dissemination literature: "experts" send information down to the community (Coleman, Katz, & Menzel, 1966; Feller, 1979; and Katz, Levin, and Hamilton, 1963; Wejnert, 2002). Classically, Ludwik Fleck described scientific findings as originating within "esoteric" circles of academic, clinical, or industrial researchers, and then flowing down to the "exoteric" circles of clinicians (Fleck, [1935]1979:111), who apply them in treating patients (Freidson [1970]1988). Indeed, this traditional top-down, bi-polar model, in which knowledge producers and users oc-

FIGURE 1. Changing Geometry of Dissemination

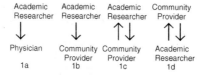

From dyadic *hierarchies* of top-down diffusion

To horizontal diffusion

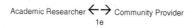

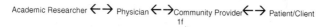

To *webs* of exchange

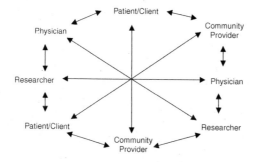

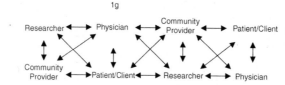

cupy separate camps, has been called the "most persistent observation in the literature on utilization" (Beyer and Trice, 1982:608).

A second limitation of the NIH approach (particularly regarding sociomedical phenomena as complex as AIDS) is that effective dissemination of information regarding early intervention and prevention requires more than merely linking physicians at one type of hospital with those at another. Channels must include, and link, community-based organizations and (as we will see) patients/clients as well–two actors traditionally ignored in dissemination models.

Third, the NIH model linked innovation only to providers serving those already in a treatment system. However, the problem of AIDS in the inner city is most severe precisely among those who are *not* in care. In these communities, the private internists who are the backbone of middle class primary care are largely absent, and the sick tend not to reach hospitals until disease is quite advanced.

Therefore, (Figure 1b) the system must extend dissemination networks past hospitals and physicians, to those in the trenches: social workers, drug counselors, health educators, community-outreach workers, the staffs of needle-exchange programs and food pantries (Indyk and Rier, 1990). The distance between such providers and the medical center is a quantum leap greater than that involved in linking community physicians to the medical center, spanning disparities of class, race, and worldview far wider than those involved in the NIH model.

In recent years, moreover, awareness of the importance of "bottom-up" flow has grown. Rather than being mere passive recipients, community providers can also be knowledge *producers* who send their insights and observations back up the line to the academics (Figure 1c). Thus, even the Centers for Disease Control and Prevention's (CDC) essentially top-down "technology transfer" model for disseminating HIV/AIDS prevention interventions from researchers to providers does call for input from "prevention service providers," community groups, and members of the target population (Kraft, Mezoff, Sogolow, Neumann, and Thomas, 2000; Kelly, Sogolow, and Neumann, 2000; see also Cotten-Oldenburg, Rosser, DeBoer, Rugg, and Carr, 2001 on the need to involve affected communities in planning prevention interventions).

But it is not enough simply to tack a bottom-up component onto this dissemination model. Both grassroots AIDS knowledge production (Indyk & Rier, 1993) and the achievements of CBOs' AIDS work belie the idea that the community necessarily constitutes the bottom. As we noted in the Introduction, there are areas in which it is the community-based provider, and not the academic researcher, who is the true expert belonging at the apex of the dissemination hierarchy (Figure 1d).

A NEW GEOMETRY OF DISSEMINATION: BEYOND BOTTOM-UP/TOP-DOWN

Better still, let us reconsider the whole concept of dissemination as a hierarchy. One major conclusion: the dissemination model must be arrayed on the *horizontal*, and no longer on the *vertical* plane. As Fawcett

(1991:625) points out, "[m]ultilevel problems require multilevel interventions." Actors at no single level or site–or type of site–command
expertise sufficient to address the full range of problems on the preven-
tion-detection-management-cure continuum. Each has his or her own
expertise, each has his or her own knowledge to contribute.

This phenomenon is captured by the concepts of "situated knowledge" (Haraway, 1991) and "local knowledge" (Geertz, 1983), which
stress that knowledge is grounded in location. Thus, actors in specific
"local" settings have their own ways of thinking and interpreting that
may differ from those of "establishment" actors. Further, they can have
access to different types of knowledge and insights. This linkage of
knowledge with location is perhaps most familiar from the parable of
the blind men and the elephant, in which blind men standing at different
spots around an elephant describe it in terms of the particular part–ear,
trunk, etc.–near which each stands.

Good (1992) has already described how international health researchers come to develop their own local knowledge so as to frame research questions and apply scientific knowledge more appropriately to
the context of their research sites. We broaden this to consider local providers and clients/patients as producers–and potential disseminators–of
knowledge and insights essential to addressing complex sociomedical
problems such as inner city AIDS. As Wynne (1991, p. 114) noted,
"Rarely, if at all, does a practical situation not need *supplementary
knowledge* in order to make scientific understanding valid and useful in
. . . context." Those with or at risk for AIDS, and the providers closest to
them, typically have personal experiences and locations in social networks that differ from those of academics. They thus see things the latter might miss. Our own work has generated phenomena such as
recovering drug addicts lecturing to medical school professors about
drug treatment efficacy.

Indeed, AIDS has already furnished a classic example of how competing world views and the differing priorities they create can produce,
not only challenges to the expertise of mainstream science, but *different*
knowledge: the debate over "gold-standard" clinical trials. By the
mid-1980s, many AIDS activists, condemning the slow pace of mainstream research on new treatments, called for liberalized clinical trials
protocols in which trials would be conducted faster, on a broader range
of experimental treatments, and would include a wider selection of
study subjects. Mainstream investigators countered that: (1) such
"quick and dirty" studies would yield results less scientifically valid than
would traditional, slower, gold-standard research; and (2) greatly liberalized

clinical trials protocols might harm study subjects. Opposing these views were AIDS activists such as Project Inform's Martin Delany and ACT-UP's Treatment and Data Committee, with a vastly different set of insight, experience, and expertise–hence, a different "definition of the situation." They argued that, since those with AIDS had a fatal, incurable disease, they needed a good answer *now*, and not a perfect answer after their death–and that, in any case, they should be allowed to decide for themselves whether to assume the risks of study participation (Epstein, 1995,1996; Indyk and Rier, 1993). They even used their unique social location and knowledge to contest credentialed scientists on their own terrain, observing that the purity of gold-standard trials was suspect. For, as they knew from anecdotal experience involving their friends and their communities, desperate clinical trial subjects would secretly violate study protocols by such stratagems as taking additional medication, or sharing medications to improve their odds of exposure to the experimental therapy, and not merely to the placebo (Epstein, 1995; Arno and Feiden, 1992:51-52, 181-82; Nussbaum, 1990).

Like the case of laymen performing and criticizing research on toxic contamination in their communities–where, too, gold-standard science was part of the dispute (Brown, 1992, 1997; Brown and Mikkelsen, 1990; Ozonoff and Boden, 1987)–this is a perfect demonstration of Latour's (1987, 1988) actor-network approach (discussed below), which views science as a political process in which competing interests and values are thrashed out, thus shaping the production of knowledge.

Also like the case of toxic-exposed communities (Brown, 1992), this is simultaneously a perfect example of how those with (or at high risk for) a disease occupy a unique social position yielding knowledge directly relevant to scientific research, which is relatively inaccessible to (credentialed) scientists. In our own work, when a client discloses to an outreach worker that people often fail to get their HIV test results because they fear deportation, both parties are adding critical information to the AIDS knowledge base–though neither may recognize it.

There are direct political and ideological implications of our broadened definition of knowledge production, our widened cast of knowledge producers. Our theoretical work, and certainly our practice–both of which seek to "represent the full array of situated knowledges" by moving beyond traditional hierarchical conceptions–can "turn up the volume on the quiet, the silent, and the silenced" (Clarke and Montini, 1993:45). Ultimately, the emergence of these voices and visions can cause, in Foucault's (1980:81) memorable phrase, an "insurrection of subjugated knowledges." In fact, Foucault explicitly expressed this in terms of local knowledge, speaking of the "reactivation of local knowledges . . . in opposition to the scientific hierarchization of knowledges and the effects intrinsic to their power. . . ." (1980: 85).

It is not that community providers–or their clients–constitute the only, or even, necessarily, the *most* legitimate sources of knowledge overall. Haraway (1991:191) has warned of the dangers of romanticizing subjugated knowledges, of regarding them as inherently, universally privileged in scientific discourse. Conversely, neither should we consider information originating from the medical center as inherently privileged. Rather, as explained in the Introduction, these differing forms of knowledge (and those producing them) *supplement* and *complement* one another.

Having seen that the "situated" character of knowledge suggests we move beyond the dissemination hierarchy entirely, we can now update our diagrams. Instead of a vertical dyad, a horizontal dyad in which the two sides are equal better reflects the valuable contribution each makes (Figure 1e). This is already recognized in the organizations literature, where Barley, Meyer, and Gash (1988:25) reject a hierarchical dyad placing academics above practitioners, in favor of a more fluid, Fleckian view of "two worlds that exist as separate but interdependent social systems. . . . [in which] the direction and degree of influence might vary from issue to issue."

But the dissemination model must be revised still further. As noted above, the greater the emphasis on prevention, the more patients need to be involved. Changing individual behavior requires the willingness to change on the part of those actually at risk. Prevention, unlike a vaccination, is neither a passive nor a one-shot process. It cannot merely be "administered" to someone. To assure their cooperation, and to insure appropriate interventions, the clients' insights are essential. For example, since interpretations and decisions regarding risk are culturally determined (Lupton, 1999; Douglas and Wildavsky, 1982), realistic interventions cannot be designed without input from the field on how clients perceive and rank various risks. Similarly, areas such as effective management of AIDS as a chronic illness or pain management require close patient involvement. Thus, as was also made clear by grassroots AIDS research (Indyk and Rier, 1993), the AIDS dissemination model must include *patients/clients* as well as community-based sociomedical providers, physicians, and researchers (Figure 1f). Traditionally, of course, as in the NIH model (Fennell and Warnecke, 1988), patients/clients were largely ignored (although, as noted above, the

CDC model has acknowledged the value of participation by target populations [Kelly, Sogolow, and Neumann, 2000]).

Since, in our linkage work, so many players (patients/clients, researchers, clinicians, administrators, etc.) contribute to dissemination and communication amongst one another, the final modification is to reject the dyad completely. Weaving together all these revisions of the classical dissemination model, we therefore speak not of dyadic *hierarchies* of top-down diffusion, but rather of matrices of relationships forming *webs* of exchange (Boggs, 1992; Huey, 1994:44; Indyk and Rier, 1993). Thus, tertiary care and community-based providers occupy not different *levels*, but different *locations* in the networks (Figure 1g). Of course, web-like circulation of information can occur only after substantial infrastructure development. Ultimately, this can result in free knowledge exchange, surmounting traditional hierarchies and boundaries, amongst "communities of practice" (Adler, Kwon, and Signer, 2003) which unite diverse players for common activities (e.g., HIV/AIDS, prevention, service and treatment).

Beyond Dissemination?

Our acceptance of the web model of dissemination leads us to Latour's (1987, 1988) actor-network model, in which distinctions between scientists (as knowledge creators) and networks of others (as knowledge users) fade. Instead, virtually all parties are seen as centrally involved in the production of knowledge (see Indyk and Rier, 1993; Rier, 1994:1544). In fact, Latour more or less rejects the whole concept of diffusion (dissemination), arguing that it presents a false image of ready-made scientific innovations being conducted, unchanged, throughout society.

Emphasizing "science-in-the-making," Latour replaces diffusion with "translation." Translation is the process through which various social actors shape, transform, package, and repackage knowledge claims so as to conform to their own interests and those of parties whose support is necessary for the claims' adoption as fact (Callon and Law, 1982; Callon, 1986). To "enroll" support, researchers will reshape their own claims to appeal to the interests of potential "allies." Conversely, they also attempt to redirect allies' interests so as to bring them in line with their own (the researchers') knowledge claims—while allies and potential allies do the same thing. It is this rough and tumble which, to Latour, *is* the production of scientific knowledge.

Even without rejecting the dissemination model, Latour's emphasis on the centrality of diverse actors is a signal contribution, with important implications for our work. Surely, AIDS activists and community providers who helped redefine both the problems and solutions in a medical center's service design and research activities, and who helped redirect the course of clinical research (who performed it, who funded it and how, how it was transmitted, what drugs were studied, what admission criteria were used in study protocols, which sub-population's problems were addressed, etc.), have become part of the scientific process. Borrowing a phrase from Collins and Pinch (1979), when community providers and activists are this intimately involved in knowledge production, *nothing unscientific is happening.*

CONCLUSION

Like the elephant in the parable described earlier, AIDS work is composed of many different parts, each with its own set of experts and expertise. Sometimes, the expertise necessary to approach an aspect of AIDS can be found in the community; other times, the answer lies with the medical center provider. For some problems, the *gemeinschaft*-style organization of the CBO is best; for others, the *gesellschaft*-style design of the medical center is needed. Managing AIDS demands recognition of the diversity of expertise. It requires, too, that the system link experts–and their institutions–and integrate their expertise. We have seen how the linkage model dictates major revisions in the composition and configuration of dissemination networks, raises basic questions about the very concept of dissemination, and suggests challenges to how we understand the border between scientists and laymen. The model summarized above recognizes that, to fulfill their respective mandates to fight AIDS in the inner city, both tertiary and community-based providers must acknowledge their interdependence (not the subordination of one to the other), and learn how to harness their complementary skills for the benefit of each other's work. Service delivery could thus be made vastly more realistic, more responsive to community problems and sensitivities, and more credible to those served.

The explicit focus of this paper has been on the circulation of knowledge and expertise throughout the system. However, another major advantage of our approach is that it allows us to tap the social contacts maintained by players at widely divergent locations within the larger social network. This is particularly clear, as noted above, when working with CBOs, whose credibility and connections within the target community are resources no less important than their unique insights into that community. However, the same principle applies to players at all the sites brought into the overall web.

By constructing the infrastructure with which to create and sustain webs of informal and formal linkages, the best of both the community-based and tertiary-care worlds can be harnessed and focused to complement one another. By cultivating a critical mass of diverse providers and patients to question, learn, and teach together, a framework is emerging through which to combat complex sociomedical challenges.

Truly, challenges such as HIV/AIDS demand the wisdom to learn from every person.

REFERENCES

Adler, P.S., Kwon, S.W., & Signer, J.M.K. (2003). The "Six West" problem: Professionals and the intraorganizational diffusion of innovations, with particular reference to the case of hospitals. URL: http://www.marshall.usc.edu/emplibrary/6west124010603.pdf

Arno, Peter S., & Feiden K.F. (1992). *Against the odds: The story of AIDS drug development, politics, & profits.* NY: Harper Collins.

Barley, S.R., Meyer, G.W., & Gash D.C. (1988). Cultures of culture: Academics, practitioners, and the pragmatics of normative control. *Administrative Science Quarterly 33,* 24-59.

Beyer, J.M., & Trice, H.M. (1982). The utilization process: A conceptual framework and synthesis of empirical findings. *Administrative Science Quarterly 27,* 591-622.

Bibeau, D.L., Howell, K.A., Rife, J.C., & Taylor, M.L. (1996). The role of a community coalition in the development of health services for the poor and uninsured. *International Journal of Health Services, 26,* 93-100.

Boggs J.P. (1992). Implicit models of social knowledge use. *Knowledge: Creation, Diffusion, Utilization, 14,* 29-62.

Brown, P. (1992). Popular epidemiology and toxic waste contamination: Lay and professional ways of knowing. *Journal of Health and Social Behavior, 33,* 267-81.

Brown, P. (1997). Popular epidemiology revisited. *Current Sociology 45*(3), 137-56.

Brown, P., & Mikkelsen, E.J. (1990). *No safe place: Toxic waste, leukemia, and community action.* Berkeley: University of California.

Callon, M. (1986). Some elements of a sociology of translation: Domestication of the scallops and the fishermen of St. Brieuc Bay. In: J. Law (Ed.), *Power, Action, and Belief [Sociological Review Monograph No. 32],* 196-233.

Callon, M., & Law, J. (1982). On interests and their transformation: Enrollment and counter-enrollment. *Social Studies of Science 12,* 615-25.

Chillag, K., Bartholow, K., Cordeiro, J., Swanson, S., Patterson, J., Stebbins, S., Woodside, C., & Francisco, S. (2002). Factors affecting the delivery of HIV/AIDS prevention programs by community-based organizations. *AIDS Education and Prevention 14*(3), 27-37.

Clarke, A. & Montini, T. (1993). The many faces of RU486: Tales of situated knowledges and technological contestations. *Science, Technology, & Human Values 18*, 42-78.

Coleman, J.S., Katz, E., & Menzel, H. (1966). *Medical Innovation: A Diffusion Study.* NY: Bobbs-Merrill.

Collins, H.M., & Pinch, T.J. (1979). The construction of the paranormal: Nothing unscientific is happening. In Wallis, R. (Ed.), *On the Margins of Science: The Social Construction of Rejected Knowledge* (pp. 237-70). Keele: University of Keele.

Cotten-Oldenburg, N.U., Rosser, B.R.S., DeBoer, J., Rugg, D.L., & Carr, P. (2001). Building strong linkages across the HIV prevention continuum: The practical lessons learned from a comprehensive evaluation effort in Minnesota. *AIDS Education and Prevention 13*(1), 29-41.

Douglas, M., & Wildavsky, A. (1982). *Risk and culture.* Berkeley: University of California Press.

Epstein, S. (1995). The construction of lay expertise: AIDS activists and the forging of credibility in the reform of clinical trials. *Science, Technology & Human Values 20*, 408-437.

Epstein, S. (1996). *Impure Science: AIDS, Activism, and the Politics of Knowledge.* Berkeley, CA: University of California Press.

Fawcett, S.B. (1991). Some values guiding community research and action. *Journal of Applied Behavioral Analysis 24*, 621-36.

Feller, I. (1979). Three coins on diffusion research. *Knowledge: Creation, Diffusion, Utilization 1*, 293-312.

Fennell, M.L., & Warnecke, R.B. (1988). *The Diffusion of Medical Innovation: An Applied Network Analysis.* NY: Plenum.

Fleck, L. [1935]1979. *Genesis and Development of a Scientific Fact* (Ed. by Trenn T.J. and Merton R.K.; tr. by Bradley F. and Trenn T.J.). Chicago: University of Chicago Press.

Foucault, M. (1980). Two lectures. pp. 78-108 in Foucault, M., *Power/knowledge: Selected interviews & other writings 1972-1977* (ed. by Gordon, C.; tr. by Gordon, C., Marshall, L., Mepham, J., and Soper, K.). NY: Pantheon.

Freidson, E. ([1970]1988). *Profession of Medicine.* Chicago: University of Chicago.

Geertz, C. (1983). *Local Knowledge.* New York: Basic Books.

Good, M.V. (1992). Local knowledge: Research capacity building in international health. *Social Science and Medicine 35*, 1359-67.

Granovetter, M. (1973). The strength of weak ties. *American Journal of Sociology, 78*, 1360-80.

Gross, M. (1993). Hospitals: Inhospitable to AIDS outreach demonstration projects for high risk pregnant women. *AIDS & Public Policy Journal 8*(3), 73-78.

Haraway, D. (1991). *Simians, Cyborgs, and Women.* New York: Routledge.

Heberle, R. (1993). Preface, p. ix in Tonnies, F., *Community and Society* (tr. by Loomis, C.P.), New Brunswick, NJ: Transaction.

Holland, J.B. (1964). Contrasting types of group relationships. pp. 208 in *Readings in Sociology*, 2nd ed. (Edited by Schuler, E.A. et al.). NY: Thomas Y. Crowell.

Huey, J. (1994). Waking up to the new economy. *Fortune*, p. 43, June 27.

Indyk, D., Boyer, A., Ellis, I. et al. (2001). Outreach as a gateway to the prevention-care-prevention continuum. National HIV Prevention Conference (Abstract #860), August 12-15.

Indyk, D., Korenblit, P., Belville, R., Barrett, E., & Rose, D. (1989). Community-based AIDS prevention and education: Linking research, resources, and community-based organizations. Presented at the Fifth International Conference on AIDS (June, Montreal).

Indyk, D., & Rier, D.A. (1990). The role of grassroots organizations in the creation, assessment and dissemination of AIDS knowledge: Overview and prognosis. Paper presented at the IV International Conference on AIDS Education. San Juan, PR, Aug. 6-8.

Indyk, D., & Rier, D.A. (1993). Grassroots AIDS knowledge: Implications for the boundaries of science and collective action. *Knowledge: Creation, Diffusion, Utilization 15*:3-43.

Indyk, D., & Rier, D.A. (this volume[a]). Wiring the HIV/AIDS system: Building interorganizational infrastructure to link people, sites, and networks. *Social Work in Health Care, 42* (3/4) 29-46.

Indyk, D., & Rier, D.A. (this volume[b]). Requisites, benefits, and challenges of sustainable HIV/AIDS system-building: Where theory meets practice. *Social Work in Health Care, 42* (3/4) 93-110.

Katz, E., Levin, M.L., & Hamilton, H. (1963). Traditions of research on the diffusion of innovation. *American Sociological Review 28*, 237-52.

Kelly, J.A., Sogolow, E.D., & Neumann, M.S., (2000). Future directions and emerging issues in technology transfer between HIV prevention researchers and community-based service providers. *AIDS Education and Prevention 12*(Supplement A), 126-41.

Kraft, J.M., Mezoff, J.S., Sogolow, E.D., Neumann, M.S., & Thomas, P.A. (2000). A technology transfer model for effective HIV/AIDS interventions: Science and practice. *AIDS Education and Prevention 12*(Supplement A), 7-20.

Latour, B. (1987). *Science in action: How to follow scientists and engineers through society.* Cambridge: Harvard University.

Latour, B. (1988). *The Pasteurization of France* (tr. by Sheridan A. and Law J.). Cambridge: Harvard University.

Litwak, E. (1985). *Helping the Elderly.* New York: Guilford Press.

Lupton, D. (Ed.) (1999). *Risk and sociocultural theory.* NY: Cambridge University Press.

Martindale, D. (1960). *The Nature and the Type of Social Theory.* Boston: Houghton Mifflin.

McKnight, J. ([1978]1990). Politicizing health care. In P. Conrad & R. Kern, (Eds.), *The Sociology of Health & Illness* (3rd ed., pp. 432-436.). New York: St. Martin's Press.

McLeroy, K.R., Bibeau, D., Steckler, A., & Glanz, K. (1988). An ecological perspective on health promotion programs. *Health Education Quarterly, 15*, 351-77.

Messeri, P., Silverstein, M., & Litwak, E. (1993). Choosing optimal support groups: A review and reformulation. *Journal of Health and Social Behavior, 34*, 122-37.

New York City Commission on HIV/AIDS (2005). Draft report [19 May]. Available from URL: *http://www.nyc.gov/html/doh/downloads/pdf/ah/ah-nychivreport.pdf* [accessed 17 July, 2005].

New York City Department of Health and Mental Hygiene (2005a). Epidemiology services, sortable statistics. Available from URL: *http://www.nyc.gov/html/doh/html/stats/stats-mortality.shtml* [accessed 14 July, 2005].

New York City Department of Health and Mental Hygiene (2005b). Community Health Profiles: The Health of East Harlem. Major Causes of Death and Hospital Admissions. Available from URL: *http://www.nyc.gov/html/doh/downloads/pdf/data/2003nhpmanh attanc.pdf* [accessed 17 July, 2005].

New York City Department of Health and Mental Hygiene (2005c). Community Health Profiles: The Health of Hunts Point and Mott Haven. Major Causes of Death and Hospital Admissions. Available from URL: *http://www.nyc.gov/html/doh/downloads/pdf/data/2003nhp-bronxd.pdf* [accessed 17 July, 2005].

New York City Department of Health and Mental Hygiene (2005d). HIV Epidemiology Program 2nd Quarter Report. Vol 3(No. 2 [April]). Available from URL: *http://www.nyc.gov/html/doh/downloads/pdf/dires/dires-2005-report-qtr2.pdf* [accessed 17 July, 2005].

Nisbet, R., & Perrin, R.G. (1977). *The Social Bond* (2nd Ed.), NY: Knopf.

Nussbaum, B. (1990). *Good Intentions.* NY: Atlantic Monthly Press.

Ozonoff, D., & Boden, L.I. (1987). Truth and consequences: Health agency responses to environmental health problems. *Science, Technology, & Human Values, 12,* 70-77.

Rier, D.A. (2004) Audience, consequence, and journal selection in toxic-exposure epidemiology. *Social Science & Medicine 59,* 1541-46.

Rotheram-Borus, M.J., Rebchook. G.M., Kelly, J.A., Adams, J., & Neumann, M.S. (2000). Bridging research and practice: Community-researcher partnerships for replicating effective interventions. *AIDS Education and Prevention, 12*(Supplement A), 49-61.

Sogolow, E.D., Kay, L.S., Doll, L.S., Neumann, M.S., Mezoff, J.S., Eke, A.N., Semaan, S., & Anderson, J.R. (2000). Strengthening HIV prevention: Application of a research-to-practice framework. *AIDS Education and Prevention, 12*(Supplement A), 21-32.

Tonnies F. ([1887]1993). *Community and Society* (tr. by Loomis, C.P.). New Brunswick, NJ: Transaction.

Wejnert, B. (2002). Integrating models of diffusion of innovations: A conceptual framework. *Annual Review of Sociology, 28,* 297-326.

Wynne, B. (1991). Knowledge in context. *Science, Technology & Human Values 16,* 111-21.

Wiring the HIV/AIDS System:
Building Interorganizational Infrastructure
to Link People, Sites, and Networks

Debbie Indyk, PhD

David A. Rier, PhD

SUMMARY. This paper presents a case example of the new "geometry of care" (Rier and Indyk, this volume), by examining selected examples from five facets of a program developed by the lead author and in operation since 1989. This program is designed to understand, build, revise, and maintain the organizational infrastructure with which to link diverse players and sites, and combine these into a web for producing, assessing, and exchanging the information needed to combat HIV/AIDS. Each example demonstrates how opportunities were exploited for developing and linking resources within and between systems of care and prevention. The program began as an iterative and systems approach to improve access of high-risk, hard-to-reach inner city New York populations to HIV/AIDS services, treatment, and research. The approach is also currently being further elaborated and applied in Argentina and India (see Boylan et al., this volume), and is adaptable to other local and global public health challenges (see Indyk & Rier, this volume).

Debbie Indyk, PhD, is affiliated with Mount Sinai School of Medicine, New York, NY. David A. Rier, PhD, is affiliated with Bar-Ilan University, Ramat-Gan, Israel.

[Haworth co-indexing entry note]: "Wiring the HIV/AIDS System: Building Interorganizational Infrastructure to Link People, Sites, and Networks." Indyk, Debbie, and David A. Rier. Co-published simultaneously in *Social Work in Health Care* (The Haworth Press, Inc.) Vol. 42, No. 3/4, 2006, pp. 29-45; and: *The Geometry of Care: Linking Resources, Research, and Community to Reduce Degrees of Separation Between HIV Treatment and Prevention* (ed: Debbie Indyk) The Haworth Press, Inc., 2006, pp. 29-45. Single or multiple copies of this article are available for a fee from The Haworth Document Delivery Service [1-800-HAWORTH, 9:00 a.m. - 5:00 p.m. (EST). E-mail address: docdelivery@haworthpress.com].

KEYWORDS. AIDS, organizations, service delivery, networks, inner city

This paper presents a case-example of the new "geometry of care" for HIV (Rier & Indyk, this volume). This work is based on the premise that each type of organization (e.g., hospital, community-based organization [CBO]) and individual (e.g., physician, scientist, patient, outreach worker) has his or her own unique perspective and expertise. These expertises need to be connected, via multi-level linkages, to enable each organization and individual to function as a distinct node in a larger web that facilitates the circulation of knowledge and the provision of coherent HIV treatment and prevention services. This paper describes how this linkage approach has been applied, via selected examples.

The enterprise we describe here is not a specific "program" or "intervention." It is something much broader and fundamental: an evolving *approach* to service design, delivery, and evaluation. In concrete terms, this approach is embodied in a long-term effort to: (1) lay the "wiring" (infrastructure) needed to promote collaboration between existing programs and services; (2) harness diverse and fluid constellations of expertise with which to design, implement, and evaluate effective programs for HIV/AIDS prevention, treatment, and sociomedical support; and (3) follow through by designing, implementing, evaluating, and revising these programs to meet emergent needs.

These ties bridge disparate settings, disciplines, and activities. They link or at least reduce degrees of separation among individuals, programs, and systems. The whole process has been an iterative, dynamic one, in which theory and practice drive one another (Indyk & Rier, this volume), and is responsive to changes in the surrounding organizational ecology. As we have applied the linkage approach, the ultimate goal has been to design and deliver improved HIV/AIDS sociomedical services to hard-to-reach populations. However, cultivating new knowledge production and dissemination channels–a "process" mainstay of this work–also constitutes its own, secondary goal.

PROMOTING LINKAGE AND COLLABORATION BETWEEN EXISTING PROGRAMS

Consistent with the assumptions of the new geometry of care (Rier & Indyk, this volume), this approach is based on the fact that providers from community-based organizations (CBOs) and academic medical centers are ideal collaborators–interdependent and complementary. The CBOs have credibility, familiarity, and access to high-risk, hard-to-reach populations. Conversely, the medical center offers advanced clinical services, technical support, and other resources important to CBOs.

As a case example, linkages between Mount Sinai Medical Center and two CBOs–Little Sisters of the Assumption Family Health Service (LSA) and Dominican Sisters Family Health Service (DSFHS)–marked one of the first fruits of this approach (Indyk, Korenblit, Belville et al., 1989; Indyk, Belville, Sweeney, Garson, 1992; Indyk, Rier, Belville et al., 1992; Indyk, Rose, Rier et al., 1993), and continue to teach us much about the potential of inter-organizational linkages. Most importantly, community-based organizations have tremendous ability to find and engage high-risk individuals. Both LSA in East Harlem and DSFHS in the South Bronx emphasize sustained, personalized sociomedical support services. These are provided in a non-threatening, "low-threshold" manner that adapts to clients' perceptions of their needs. This approach has won them the trust of their high-risk clientele, usually among the most elusive to the system. Initial engagement for one specific problem is a gateway to managing other issues: as in peeling an onion, new layers of problems are revealed with time. Deeper knowledge of clients' circumstances, in turn, makes screening, follow-up, and service design far more effective.

The CBOs' orientation towards intimate primary attachments fills a particular void in the inner city, where family ties have often been strained by poverty, substance abuse, incarceration, violence, and illness. These CBOs feature intensive involvement with families, and help fill needs left unmet by missing primary support ties. These even include such services as knocking on a mother's door every morning to ensure that she's gotten her children ready for school, or that she's taking her tuberculosis medication.

At the same time, CBOs benefit greatly from collaboration with major medical centers, which can offer access to a variety of services traditionally beyond their reach. For example, CBOs normally lack ready access to advanced or specialized medical care and clinical research, and require staff education regarding AIDS and its state-of-the-art prevention and treatment. Through the linkage approach, CBO providers can receive such training. Mount Sinai providers supply community providers with extensive grant development, in-services, data management, evaluation, service design and implementation, and other technical support. Joint grant development has proved particularly successful. Mount Sinai also offers linkages to clinical and research resources otherwise unavailable to community providers. In turn, the community-based agencies provide academic institutions with access to critical masses of individuals who are traditionally underrepresented in clinical trials research, and who can be linked to community-based providers through the web of linkages established. However, we have found that the recruitment of individuals to trials requires the establishment of more complex 'wiring' to support the development of community-level and individual interest, trust and commitment to clinical research (Indyk, Rier, Belville, Sacks, Chusid, Sweeney, & Garson, 1992).

The challenge of recruiting individuals to trials is even greater today, since the majority of drug trials for chronic conditions like HIV are needed to demonstrate relative life extending benefits rather than life-saving treatment. Community-based providers can provide a critical doorway to clinical trials. In fact DSFHS currently includes, as 'standard of care' for its HIV-infected clients, education about clinical trials, in general, and, in particular, about HIV trials available in the community. Implementing and sustaining this standard requires ongoing staff development to train all service providers to integrate this education into care plans. It also requires an agency clinician to develop the infrastructure with external agencies with which to keep abreast of current and emerging research. Over time, providers at DSFHS have become involved in generating research questions, and work closely with academic researchers to establish formal research projects.

In this way, the benefits of collaboration accrue both to CBO and medical center. CBOs can also disseminate their unique observations across multiple boundaries to reach both clients in need of care and the medical center, as well as to refer clients for treatment and services at the medical center. In so doing, they have helped the medical center fulfill its mandate of serving those most in need (and traditionally underserved). They also offer the detailed knowledge of the community without which effective interventions are scarcely possible even to design, much less execute.

Linkage agreements between CBOs and the medical center have created bi-directional referrals between the community and medical center. The fruits include concrete new services reaching an underserved population who traditionally entered the health care system only through the Emergency Department. Early collaborative resource development secured funds which enabled LSA and DSFHS to expand their capacity to serve approximately 20 "walk-ins" daily needing shelter, food or entitlement. In addition to responding to these emergent needs, this doorway was used to develop and incorporate vulnerability and risk-assessments. These became components of their intake for *all* walk-ins, while the same doorway also has been used to support engagement and retention in supportive services, follow-up, and case management.

Advances in the treatment of HIV/AIDS since the advent of Highly Active Antiretroviral Therapy (HAART) medication in the late 1990s fueled a need for further changes in the geometry of care. During the early 1990s, the locus of care shifted from acute care settings to hospice care and the community, requiring primarily bi-directional referrals. By the turn of century, it became clear that new approaches were needed to find, engage and support individuals along the continuum of HIV risk and disease.

One innovation has been the elaboration of outreach as a methodology for engagement. Originally, DSFHS defined outreach as offering HIV/AIDS services to their existing client base and walk-ins, who came in search of various social and advocacy services. Today, this is considered "*in*-reach" to existing clients. *Outreach* now means reaching those not yet involved with DSFHS, and those not yet engaged at all. Thus, outreach programs have been designed to locate underserved clients, literally, "where they're at": near the drug treatment clinic, in the Ob-Gyn ward, on the street corner (Belville, Indyk, Astor, and Sweeney, 1993). For example, many senior citizens are HIV-infected, but are neither diagnosed nor in sustained care. DSFHS is establishing linkages with senior centers, not only to provide education and testing, but to support medication management, counseling, and retention in care.

Linkages are also being developed with other CBOs who provide similar community-based services for special needs populations, so as to leverage community capacity. For example, social service providers working with the severely mentally ill have few structural linkages to HIV service providers. It is often through bottom-up linkages that infrastructure is developed. DSFHS is cultivating other CBOs, those with

.engaged clients but lacking the capacity to provide HIV/AIDS services, as sites for collaboration. These other CBOs provide access to their hard-to-reach-populations, and DSFHS offers vital HIV/AIDS services. DSFHS is thus replicating with other CBOs what Mount Sinai has built with it, demonstrating the potential self-sustainability and self-perpetuation of the work.

An important aspect of DSFHS' work is developing programs to harness the human potential of their own clients to work with the community. After a pilot program trained eight clients of its Mother's Group to do street, home-based, and agency outreach, a Peer Outreach group was formed. This group has created peer educators who help reach out to nearly 8,000 community residents. Once reached, these residents are given health education, and encouraged to enter the DSFHS network of services for testing, counseling, prevention, and treatment (Indyk, Boyer, Pilgrim et al., 2001). DSFHS developed an onsite HIV counseling and testing program in 2003 and expanded it in 2004, together with off-site social work services to further extend its reach to those unaware of their status, as well as to those who are aware but not in care. The special insights and expertise of its clients are also tapped through its Client Advisory Group (CAG). The CAG clients: formulated their own mission statement; defined position descriptions for members; advocated for, planned, and executed a focus group program for teens and their parents; and participated in other program planning. CAG members receive stipends for assisting with outreach and health fairs. Members attend national conferences, and are presenting at local conferences (Little, 2003).

HARNESSING EXPERTISE, BUILDING KNOWLEDGE

Often, one of the most difficult features of this approach to infrastructure building and collaboration is the lack of specific forums and structures within which diverse actors can share their expertise. Below, we outline components of the infrastructure created to provide such forums, and briefly review their outcomes.

Community Case Rounds

The HIV Community Case Rounds group (Indyk & Wade, 1992) was developed and maintained by several stakeholders (such as the Mount Sinai HIV education program, and the local HIV Care Network) to address cross-system coordination challenges. Community-based providers were confronting complex problems during their clients' post-hospital discharge period. These rounds were initiated to bring together community- and hospital-based front-line providers, who had traditionally represented very different camps. The group generated both monthly inter-agency rounds at the community network level and ongoing community-based case study analysis. Participants included community-based providers (such as drug treatment counselors, social workers, housing specialists, and nurses) together with academic physicians and other medical school faculty. Through this framework, providers from vastly different backgrounds and work settings shared in presenting cases *as colleagues.* Efforts were made to enroll new participants so that case rounds remained relevant despite shifts in the epidemic.

These and other case rounds that they generated have been a vehicle for diverse providers collectively to identify and interpret new or changing patterns. From such a process, consensus has emerged, and formed the basis for joint action. Currently, multi-system case rounds are critical for the improved engagement, retention, and management of individuals with multiple co-morbidities, including advanced chronic diseases, mental illness, addictions, and homelessness.

In uniting for the common purpose of exchanging insights and information with which to combat HIV/AIDS, these providers form a multidisciplinary "community of practice" (Wenger, 1998; Adler, Kwon, Signer, 2003; Housego, 2002). They thus blur and help surmount traditional functional boundaries between researchers and practitioners, between physicians and other providers, and between community and medical center. Simultaneously, they help bypass status hierarchies that normally accompany such boundaries. Part of the challenge (and opportunity) has been in helping providers realize their potential power as creators and assessors of such new knowledge.

CDC Prevention Planning Group (PPG)

Another important linkage mechanism has been fostered through the New York State and New York City Prevention Planning Groups (PPGs). In the early 1990s, the Centers for Disease Control and Prevention (CDC) mandated that each jurisdiction receiving federal prevention dollars create a representative coalition of participants for intensive, sustained work to apply data and knowledge to HIV harm reduction. Through this forum, consumers (citizens, clients, and patients), grassroots providers, academic researchers, government agencies, communities, and the systems behind them are linked structurally and functionally. The first author identified this group as a vehicle for achieving bottom-up, top-down linkages, and served five years as a member of its Executive Committee and two years as the New York State co-chair. As co-chair she drew on the framework described above to foster opportunities through the monthly Executive Committee meetings, population-focused committees such as the Women's, Substance Users, and Men Who Have Sex with Men Committees, as well as through bi-monthly full committee meetings to share the respective insights and experiences of these diverse participants. The challenge was to use this infrastructure to produce, harness, assess, transmit, and apply new knowledge about behavioral prevention interventions.

This process was used to identify service needs and then to help formulate the services and policies necessary. For example, one Women's Committee member's front-line experiences as a nurse practitioner, combined with the emerging research literature, led that committee to the early recognition that preventing (primary prevention) or treating (secondary prevention) sexually transmitted diseases (STDs) can be a form of primary prevention of HIV. Thus, the Women's Committee (with DI as chair) began pushing for the integration of STD and HIV prevention, education, and treatment. Despite encountering strong resistance, the group achieved some successes to date (yet, a decade later, continues to surmount organizational, administrative, and attitudinal barriers to this integration). Another insight arising from the PPG work has been recognition of the need to apply behavioral science findings, such as the "stages of change" theory (Prochaska & DiClimente, 1986), to the design of HIV/AIDS programs (Indyk, Coury-Doniger, Grosz et al., 1997). This insight has been integrated into the authors' work to understand and explain impediments to effecting change at the system, provider, and client levels.

Overall, these groups bring two particular benefits. First, their regional scope affords greater "reach," permitting linkage of networks and systems, rather than of individual programs or sites. Second, this "bird's eye" scope, combined with the comparative clout of PPG members, permits both greater coordination and the reshaping of funding patterns to direct more resources to linkage activities.

HIV/Substance Abuse Working Group

The origins of this group lay in the East Harlem Community Health Committee (EHCHC), a consortium of disparate community-based agencies and units from several hospitals working together to coordinate and integrate public health action in East Harlem. From an original Substance Abuse working group in the early 1990s, the HIV focus evolved into an additional component that was based at Mount Sinai. Eventually, there developed a critical mass of professionals interested in substance abuse and its connections with HIV/AIDS (thus forming another community of practice).

This group's diverse core was composed of the Mount Sinai AIDS Center Health Education Coordinator, social workers, nurse clinicians, nurse practitioners, staff from several methadone programs, drug treatment counselors, and recovering addicts. Diversity existed even within given fields. Among drug treatment professionals, for example, those advocating residential treatment would rarely otherwise have communicated–much less collaborated–with their colleagues favoring the methadone maintenance approach and eclectic and lower threshold (harm reduction) approaches.

Recognizing that actors at all positions of the system have their own particular expertise, this group viewed current and former drug users as the experts on many issues related to HIV and substance abuse. In fact, as part of this group's activities, a panel of recovering addicts gave a series of presentations on the efficacy of various treatments in HIV-positive addicts. At the end, the presenters answered questions from the audience, which included academic physicians. The participation of these panelists, who have all gone from being clients to heads of programs, helped reframe HIV management to address addiction problems. As experts on treatment they have become authorities, first for current drug users on the street and then for academic physicians as well. Only through interdisciplinary linkages is such information transmission possible: These diverse providers would never have met in traditionally-organized settings.

As Granovetter's (1973) work on the strength of weak ties would predict, it is precisely *because* contact between such disparate providers is rare that these bridging devices yield rich benefits.

Weekly AIDS Center Conference Series

This conference series (500 sessions over 13 years) brought together diverse medical center and community providers to share, learn, and network. Regular participants included physicians, patients, drug counselors, researchers, administrators, and others. A wide range of Mount Sinai departments have been represented, from Housekeeping to Liver Transplant. Similarly, over 20 community agencies participated regularly, representing almost all of the major primary care providers, as well as government and grassroots organizations. From 1990-2003, these sessions were held at the medical center and widely promoted through monthly mailings, faxes, and postings. Together, participants explored topics ranging from updates on basic and clinical science research to discussions of emotional coping styles, clinical management, clinical trials, community organizing, ethical dilemmas, policy developments, and education/prevention issues. For years, the weekly seminar played a vital role for a wide range of providers, for whom this was one of their only methods of keeping abreast of AIDS developments, and of meeting other providers confronting AIDS.

As other channels developed to offer providers access to the growing number of HIV resources available locally and on the Internet, conferences were web-cast and archived online, creating a body of material that can be accessed real-time or at the user's convenience.

Mount Sinai AIDS Center Clinical Education Initiative (CEI)

The Clinical Education Initiative (CEI), funded by the NYS Department of Health (AIDS Institute), was developed as a responsive community exchange model for training clinicians in HIV/AIDS work. The program reached community-based providers "where they're at" geographically, as well as with respect to their knowledge base, experience, and comfort level in counseling, testing, diagnosing and managing HIV disease. It supplied level-appropriate and updated clinical practice information. Outreach of medical center staff and clinicians to community providers and their support staff helped to reduce degrees of separation among HIV providers practicing in remote settings and community-based providers unwilling or unable to come to sessions conducted in the medical center. In many ways, the outreach methodology was informed by outreach to hard-to-reach HIV infected clients. By going to their sites, on their turf, it was easier to establish trust and a collegial relationship with community providers at various stages of engagement in the provision of HIV care and prevention.

In turn, center-based sessions provided "inreach" opportunities for confronting emerging issues (such as substance use, behavioral research, and co-morbidities) in sessions that would not normally attract center-based clinicians. Once a critical mass of practitioners working in the drug treatment arena became comfortable functioning as a 'community of practice' and began also to attend–and integrate with clinicians attending–the weekly HIV conferences, they began to share their experiences and be recognized by academic clinicians and researchers as experts.

The various educational forum modalities developed and sustained through this program included: hospital-based case rounds; continuing HIV/AIDS education and training; a weekly lecture series; community-wide case rounds; community-wide workshops; a community network of providers; patient forums; and a clearinghouse for assessing and disseminating emerging knowledge. CEI embodied the core assumption of all our work: that formal new scientific knowledge and the unique insights of front-line providers are both critical to the success of AIDS care, education, and prevention. Thus, when community providers had inpatient preceptorships, they learned about HIV management, but *also* shared their community-based front-line experiences and knowledge of the patient with the hospital-based specialist: Each informed the other.

The CEI program created pathways through which to link what are normally considered "bottom-up" and "top-down" forms of knowledge transfer. It thus facilitated transmission of new information: across systems of care and prevention; from academic center to community settings; and from community providers detecting and treating previously-undiagnosed disease to HIV specialists in tertiary settings. Overall, the CEI supported linkages among disciplines within the medical center, communication among the local community-based organizations, and local and cosmopolitan networks of researchers, practitioners, patients, and educators. The CEI model has proven flexible enough to adapt new knowledge, useful for sharing information, and important in training researchers and care providers in different disciplines.

DESIGNING NEW PROGRAMS

Health Bridge: Frontline Service, Frontline Knowledge Exchange

The basic goal of our application of the linkage approach is to bring sociomedical HIV/AIDS services to the hard-to-reach. Though Mount Sinai operates a Designated AIDS Center offering state-of-the-art clinical management of HIV/AIDS, many of those most needing its services never reach its doors. Consider HIV+ residents of Single Room Occupancy hotels (SROs) in Manhattan's Upper West Side. Lacking their own homes, these residents are placed in SROs by the City, but generally lack ready access to even basic medical services. Members of this high-risk, transient, hard-to-reach population: live alone; often lack fundamental social and family supports; are frequently in denial about their HIV status; experience daily life as threatening and difficult; lack adequate nutrition; are likely to be active substance abusers; are intimidated by the rules and requirements of traditional medical providers; and often suffer from co-morbidities, including diabetes, asthma, or mental illness. Access to such a population would turn SROs into strategic sites to engage precisely those least likely to be reached by traditional services (London, Indyk, Clark et al., 1998). Recognizing this, a medical school professor and a physician assistant created Health Bridge, an innovative program designed to bring primary care to this profoundly marginalized population.

Given the complexity of these clients' sociomedical problems, and their often strained history of relations with the conventional medical system, Health Bridge emphasizes a gradual, consumer-oriented approach. This "low-threshold," non-threatening method permits clients to pursue only those services for which they are ready at a given moment. Whenever possible, services are delivered onsite at the SROs. These include: immunizations, lab tests, urgent medical care, psychiatric referrals, care coordination counseling, health education, and facilitated referral and linkage to primary and specialty medical care and social services. Care coordinators assist clients by setting the appointments and arranging escorts to navigate clients through the system.

A consistent feature of this work is the labor-intensive effort to identify, engage, encourage, and monitor clients. First-level contact is generally made by a clinician knocking on SRO doors to offer on-site medical care. Special attention is given to meeting what clients initially define as their immediate needs, such as food. Another route consists of periodic "public health sweeps" in which staff offer clients services such as vaccination, blood pressure or hearing testing, or vitamins. Once providers and clients are accustomed to one another, clients may eventually be ready for the next step (see Boyer & Indyk, this volume). Health Bridge then links them to a wider range of ancillary services, such as detoxification. Finally, clients prepared to receive their primary care in traditional settings are referred to a full range of medical services, as well as drug counseling and adherence workshops, at Mount Sinai. Apart from arranging for, reminding clients about, and escorting them to such visits, staff also provide "Metro Cards" for mass transportation and meal vouchers, if necessary, in order to further smooth the process.

One interesting pilot project offered by Health Bridge is its Breakfast Club. Clients beginning HIV/AIDS treatment are given meal vouchers for a local diner where they meet regularly over breakfast to discuss their questions, fears, and experiences about treatment. More than a support group, this forum is also a tool with which staffers tap the critical "local knowledge" (Geertz, 1983) and expertise of their clientele in understanding the realities of HIV/AIDS treatment.

The core Health Bridge team is composed of: a part-time physician; a physician assistant who serves as clinical coordinator; a medical assistant who manages lab tests and sets up clinical appointments, reminders, and escorts for clients ready to engage in traditional clinical care; and four care coordinators who offer crisis and harm-reduction case management services such as nutritional support and referrals to housing, medical care, and drug treatment. A critical component of the program is a sophisticated data system that provides reports that staff use to plan daily activities and follow-up (Indyk & Indyk, this volume). Participant observation of Health Bridge team meetings indicates that there exists a true team approach. Rather than a traditional model in which expertise and authority are hierarchically ascribed by educational credentials, Health Bridge–reflecting the theoretical insights at the heart of the entire linkage enterprise (Rier & Indyk, this volume)–approaches them as situation- or location-specific. Thus, the physician and medical school professor on the team are deeply attentive to the insights of the outreach worker into the day-to-day problems (such as gastric upset, missing Medicaid cards) clients face in beginning and managing their medical treatment.

A major focus of Health Bridge work is helping its outreach staff appreciate their value as creators, assessors, and disseminators of new knowledge. Their close familiarity with the daily lives of Health Bridge clients uniquely positions them to identify and interpret emerging health risks and service needs. Traditionally, the system has rarely tapped the insights of such individuals. If these workers are able to redefine their traditional role by learning systematically to process and transmit their insights, they contribute immeasurably to the HIV/AIDS knowledge base. Health Bridge taps their insights through such devices as twice-weekly case conferences. In fact, the Breakfast Club demonstrates that this process can be extended to clients, themselves. These mechanisms for eliciting "real-time" information make Health Bridge a vital field surveillance unit for tracking changes in the high-risk community, and in the course of HIV/AIDS.

Overall, Health Bridge has served as a running laboratory for what we can do in the community to improve services for those least engaged. In the past six years, Health Bridge has served close to 800 SRO residents. Over 350 of these individuals were linked to primary care services, 270 to inpatient services, and 200 to specialty care. In an average month, it maintains an active roster of about 130 clients. Demonstrating its strategic role in reaching the hard-to-reach, Health Bridge referrals currently account for one-quarter of Mount Sinai Medical Center's inpatient census and ten percent of its clinic visits.

Argentina as a Strategic Site for Research and Training in HIV Knowledge Transfer

Argentina's health care system is generally high-quality and well-organized. Yet, reflecting the nation's wide internal economic disparities, most patients outside the private clinical system of the large urban centers receive no diagnosis, treatment, or care unless and until the individual takes the initiative, and seeks care for symptomatic illness. Applied to diseases such as HIV/AIDS, this means a near absence of prevention, screening, or early identification of those infected. The exceptions are limited, and exist due to HIV/AIDS pioneers and activists. While there are many HIV/AIDS scientists in Argentina, HIV prevention across the different disciplines does not currently exist as an active, collaborative enterprise.

Mount Sinai, in concert with other institutions in the US and Argentina, has developed and implemented an approach to help meet this need. This approach, exporting and extending the work done in New York City, involves building infrastructure with which to develop a sustained training system to support the creation and integration of new prevention knowledge. The program creates mechanisms to support the cultivation of research capacity at the individual and system level, and draws trainees from a wide range of disciplines and sites. In particular, it goes beyond the hospital, to build linkages to parties better positioned to reach and serve people at earlier stages of the disease cycle.

The research training program offers various types of multi-disciplinary training in seven settings within the Buenos Aires community. Topics include: (1) biomedical prevention research; (2) behavioral and sociomedical prevention research; (3) data management and analysis; and (4) translational research that can draw upon basic, biologic, and behavioral science. The model is a "bottom-up/top-down" approach that links research training and resources to strategic community-based settings, thus promoting circulation of insights among disparate locations of the overall health system.

Ultimately, the goal is to establish and maintain a multi-site, multi-level network of providers and sites, to promote communication and collaboration. This network is being modeled using lessons learned in working with the CDC Community Prevention Planning Groups. As envisioned in our original application, the grant was to lead to the development of multiple new programs, policy changes, and new collaborative initiatives among the faculty and trainees (Indyk, Gurtman, Stephens et al., 1998). To date, the first cycle of funding (2000-2005), has spawned 53 short- and long-term research training opportunities for Argentine practitioners.

CONCLUSION

The basic achievement of this work has been to extend, via linkages between disparate sectors in the fight against AIDS, sociomedical HIV/AIDS services to high-risk, hard-to-reach inner city residents. Provider to provider, program to program, network to network linkages are established, maintained, and revised to meet emerging needs. Simultaneously, the functions of prevention and care, and of education, service delivery, and research, are bridged. Frontline, community-based providers are linked with academic clinicians and researchers. Directly and indirectly, each of the above is better linked to clients and patients. In so doing, we help surmount barriers of hierarchy and status that in the traditional system impede two-way information transfer and cooperation.

Each of the programs described embodies part of the central insights behind this approach as a whole. Some are important mainly to initiate contact between actors (individuals or organizations) from disparate locations and functions within the system. Such programs constitute "wiring," the linkages that facilitate the sustained, multi-disciplinary communication and collaboration so vital for further work. Other programs are best seen as end products, directly fulfilling our goal of improving HIV/AIDS sociomedical services to those most at risk.

All of these programs constitute concrete evidence for the key insight behind the new geometry of care: Actors at all points in the system possess expertise vital to tackling sociomedical challenges as complex as the HIV/AIDS epidemic.

REFERENCES

Adler, P.S., Kwon, S.W., & Signer, J.M.K. (2003). The "Six West" problem: Professionals and the intraorganizational diffusion of innovations, with particular reference to the case of hospitals. URL: *http://www.marshall.usc.edu/emplibrary/6west124010603.pdf* [accessed 18 July, 2005].

Belville, R., Indyk, D., Astor, B., & Sweeney, M. (1993). Risk assessment and reduction among high-risk minorities through sustained outreach and follow-up. Poster presented at the IX International Conference on AIDS, Berlin, Germany.

Belville, R., Indyk, D., Shapiro, V., Dewart, T., Moss, J.Z., Gordon, G., & LaChapelle, S. (1992). The community as a strategic site for refining high risk perinatal assessments and interventions. *Social Work in Health Care 16*(1), 5-19.

Boyer, A., & Indyk, D. (this volume). Shaping garments of care: Maximizing tools for adherence. *Social Work in Health Care, 42*(3/4), 149-164.

Centers for Disease Control and Prevention. (2001). Interventions for HIV Positive Individuals. In: *HIV Prevention Strategic Plan through 2005.*

Geertz, C. (1983). Local Knowledge. New York: Basic Books.

Granovetter, M. (1973). The strength of weak ties. *American Journal of Sociology, 78,* 1360-80.

Housego, S. (2002, December). Boundary crossing in a community of practice. Proceedings of the Annual Conference, Australasian Society for Computers in Learning in Tertiary Education, Auckland, New Zealand. URL: *http://www.ascilite.org.au/conferences/auckland02/proceedings/papers/121.pdf* [accessed 18 July, 2005].

Indyk, D., Belville, R., Gordon, G., Dewart, T., & LaChapelle, S. (1993). A community-based approach to HIV case management: Systematizing the unmanageable. *Social Work, 38,* 380-87.

Indyk, D., Rier, D., Belville, R., Sacks, H., Chusid, E., Sweeney, M., & Garson, J. (1992). Community partnerships for service, education, and AIDS clinical trials. Paper presented at the 120th Annual Meeting of the American Public Health Association, Washington, D.C.

Indyk, D., Belville, R., Sweeney, M., & Garson, J.R. (1992, July). A community partnership model of AIDS intervention for an inner-city population in an environment of scarce resources. Paper presented at an invitational workshop at the Fourth International Conference on Social Work and AIDS, Washington, D.C.

Indyk, D., Boyer, A., Pilgrim, A., Farrington, C., Sweeney, M., & Strauss, D. (2001, August). Outreach as a gateway to the prevention-care-prevention continuum: Results of a continuous quality approach to program, staff and data development and evaluation. Paper presented at the National HIV Prevention Conference, Atlanta, GA (Abstract #860).

Indyk, D., Coury-Doniger, P., Grosz, J., Pruden, S., Jordan, S., Kaudeyr, K., Edwards, T., Klein, S., & Stevens, P.C. (1997, July). HIV Prevention: Applying 'Stages of Change' theory to accelerate bottom-up and top-down prevention knowledge production and technology transfer. Paper presented at the Public Health Conference on Records and Statistics and the National Committee on Vital and Health Statistics, Washington, D.C.

Indyk, D., Gurtman, A., Stephens, P.C., Reboredo, G., Ballve, M., Cahn, P., Casetti, I., Szarlardi, M., & Bologna, R. (1998, July). Planning to change and changing to plan technology transfer: Applying lessons learned from prevention planning in the U.S. to inform efforts in Argentina. Paper presented at the XII International AIDS Conference, Geneva, Switzerland [Abstract #43177].

Indyk, D., Korenblit, P., Belville, R., Barrett, E., & Rose, D. (1989, June). Community-based AIDS prevention and education: Linking research, resources, and community-based organizations. Paper presented at the V International Conference on AIDS, Montreal, Canada.

Indyk, D., & Rier, D.A. (1990, August). The role of grassroots organizations in the creation, assessment and dissemination of AIDS knowledge: Overview and prognosis. Paper presented at the IV International Conference on AIDS Education. San Juan, Puerto Rico.

Indyk, D., & Rier, D.A. (this volume). Requisites, benefits, and challenges of sustainable HIV/AIDS system-building: Where theory meets practice. *Social Work in Health Care, 42*(3/4), 93-110.

Indyk, D., Rier, D.A., Belville, R., Sacks, H., Chusid, E., Sweeney, M., & Garson, J. (1992, November). Community partnerships for service, education, and AIDS clinical trials. Paper presented at the 120th Annual American Public Health Association Meeting, Washington, D.C.

Indyk, D., Rose, D., Rier, D., Belville, R., Dewart, T., & Korenblit, P. (1993). Linking resources, education, research and community-based organizations: A status report. Paper presented at the IX International Conference on AIDS, Berlin, Germany.

Indyk, D., & Wade, K. (1992). Integrating community and hospital-based case management. *FOCUS: A Guide to AIDS Research and Counseling 7*(10):1-5.

Indyk, L. & Indyk, D (this volume). Collecting data along the continuum of care and prevention: A continuous quality improvement approach. *Social Work in Health Care, 42*(3/4), 47-60.

Little, W. (2003, January). Interdisciplinary Theoretical Perspectives on HIV Adherence. Patient Forum, Mount Sinai Medical Center, New York.

London, K., Indyk, D., Clark, J., Stancliff, S., Lee, A., & Nardi, S. (1998, June). Results of a clinical outreach to HIV infected individuals living in SRO hotels. Paper presented at the XII International AIDS Conference, Geneva, Switzerland [Abstract #12447].

Prochaska, J.O., & DiClemente, C.C. (1986). Toward a comprehensive model of change. In W.R. Miller and N. Heather (Eds.), *Treating addictive behaviors: Processes of change* (pp. 3-27). NY: Plenum Press.

Rier, D.A., & Indyk, D. (this volume). The rationale of interorganizational linkages to connect multiple sites of expertise, knowledge production, and knowledge transfer: An example from HIV/AIDS services for the inner city. *Social Work in Health Care, 42*(3/4), 9-28.

Wenger, E. (1998). *Communities of practice: Learning, meaning, and identity.* New York: Cambridge University Press.

Collecting Data Along the Continuum of Prevention and Care: A Continuous Quality Improvement Approach

Leonard Indyk, PhD
Debbie Indyk, PhD

SUMMARY. For the past 14 years, a team of applied social scientists and system analysts has worked with a wide variety of Community-Based Organizations (CBO's), other grassroots agencies and networks, and Medical Center departments to support resource, program, staff and data development and evaluation for hospital- and community-based programs and agencies serving HIV at-risk and affected populations.

A by-product of this work has been the development, elaboration and refinement of an approach to Continuous Quality Improvement (CQI) which is appropriate for diverse community-based providers and agencies. A key component of our CQI system involves the installation of a sophisticated relational database management and reporting system (DBMS) which is used to collect, analyze, and report data in an iterative process to provide feedback among the evaluators, agency administra-

Leonard Indyk, PhD, is affiliated with BRADLI Associates, Teaneck, NJ. Debbie Indyk, PhD, is affiliated with Mount Sinai School of Medicine, New York, NY.

[Haworth co-indexing entry note]: "Collecting Data Along the Continuum of Prevention and Care: A Continuous Quality Improvement Approach." Indyk, Leonard, and Debbie Indyk. Co-published simultaneously in *Social Work in Health Care* (The Haworth Press, Inc.) Vol. 42, No. 3/4, 2006, pp. 47-60; and: *The Geometry of Care: Linking Resources, Research, and Community to Reduce Degrees of Separation Between HIV Treatment and Prevention* (ed: Debbie Indyk) The Haworth Press, Inc., 2006, pp. 47-60. Single or multiple copies of this article are available for a fee from The Haworth Document Delivery Service [1-800-HAWORTH, 9:00 a.m. - 5:00 p.m. (EST). E-mail address: docdelivery@haworthpress.com].

tion and staff. The database system is designed for two purposes: (1) to support the agency's administrative internal and external reporting requirements; (2) to support the development of practice driven health services and early intervention research. The body of work has fostered a unique opportunity for the development of exploratory service-driven research which serves both administrative and research needs. *[Article copies available for a fee from The Haworth Document Delivery Service: 1-800-HAWORTH. E-mail address: <docdelivery@haworthpress.com> Website: <http://www.HaworthPress.com> © 2006 by The Haworth Press, Inc. All rights reserved.]*

KEYWORDS. Continuous Quality Improvement, relational database, capacity building

For the past 14 years, a team of applied social scientists and system analysts has worked with a wide variety of Community-Based Organizations (CBO's), other grassroots agencies and networks, and medical center departments to support resource, program, staff and data development and evaluation for hospital- and community-based programs and agencies serving HIV at-risk and affected populations. The collaboration has strengthened infrastructures within and between systems of care and prevention, developed sustained educational forums, and provided consultation and sustained funding streams for 10 CBO's, 3 coalitions, and 7 hospital programs linking Medical Center and grassroots agencies and networks (see Indyk & Rier, this volume).

In working with each of these organizations, we have found that in order to properly analyze and evaluate the current activities and populations served, and to recommend comprehensive future programs, staff need data. Indeed, the combination of the detailed reporting requirements of various service reimbursers combined with the data-driven requirements of virtually every potential funding organization (both government and private) has forced CBO's to duplicate, on a shoestring budget, what a medical center MIS department provides.

A by-product of this work has been the development, elaboration and refinement of an approach to Continuous Quality Improvement (CQI) which is appropriate for diverse community-based providers and agencies (Indyk & Indyk, 1995). This work is based on the premise that the same sophisticated tools and thinking commonly used by large institutions can be used to great advantage by small, often complex CBO's. A key component of our CQI system involves the installation of a sophisticated relational database management and reporting system (DBMS) which is used to collect, analyze, and report data in an iterative process involving frequent meetings to provide feedback among the evaluators, agency administration and staff. The database system is designed for two purposes: (1) to support the agency's administrative internal and external reporting requirements (streamlining record-keeping and minimizing duplication of data-collection effort); and (2) to support the development of practice driven health services and early intervention research. The body of work has fostered a unique opportunity for the development of exploratory service-driven research which serves both administrative and research needs.

This work represents a critical piece of infrastructure for the instantiation of the new geometry of care (Rier & Indyk, this volume). In that context, this paper presents mini case-studies of how data systems have been developed and maintained to support and expand webs of interorganizational linkages and grassroots efforts through three very different projects. The first is: Dominican Sisters Family Health Service (DSFHS) located within the Mott Haven section of the South Bronx in New York City, a certified multi-service, home-based health and social service program. DSFHS provides coordinated medical, psychosocial and related support services and linkages to research, to women, children and families living with and affected by HIV/AIDS. The communities served by DSFHS represent the most vulnerable individuals and families in New York City. The population of the seven zip codes is reported to be 312,630 residents. These zip code areas are also referred to as Mott Haven, Hunts Point, Highbridge and Morrisania. It is important to note that though the agency outreaches to the seven zip codes, most of its services are provided to those in the Mott Haven and Highbridge sections (zip codes 10452, 10454 and 10455). The agency serves over 3,500 individuals belonging to 2,000 families each year. We have worked with the agency for 14 years and during this time, we have helped the agency amass data on 9,000 families, 21,000 individuals and over 42,000 visits since 1992. The second site is Mount Sinai's NYS designated AIDS Center, the Jack Martin Fund Clinic (JMFC). Mount Sinai has been a designated AIDS Center since 1990. Although the JMFC is an outpatient clinic, its clinical staff also cares for all Mount Sinai inpatients with an AIDS diagnosis. Over the last 14 years our database system tracked the activities of over 8,500 patients who made 130,000 clinic visits to the JMFC and had 14,000 hospital admissions. A very large suite of reports were generated monthly, quarterly and annually and distributed and utilized by JMFC administration and clinical staff.

The third project, Health Bridge (HB), is a six-year old hospital-based clinical outreach program serving over 750 HIV infected patients who are being housed by New York City's HIV/AIDS Service Administration (HASA), in Single-Room-Occupancy facilities (SRO's). A description of the processes and content of our CQI model at each of these sites illustrates many of the lessons we have learned over the past 14 years, and traces the evolution of data systems that truly support collaboration between traditional academic medical centers and more innovative, community-based approaches to HIV prevention and treatment. In understanding the model that follows, it is important to note that the first step in approaching each agency we have worked with is to make a detailed analysis of the organization's structure, purpose, staffing, client base, and funding sources. One of the most critical questions which is asked of the agency's administration and staff during the initial assessment is "what information and reports do you need from the database management system (DBMS)?" It might appear that by starting with the end product (reports) we are putting the cart before the horse–asking about end-products before determining what data the agency is currently collecting. However, over time, and in every type of setting, one of the predictable outcomes of on-going feedback to staff and continued staff input has been the need to expand the type and extent of data collected in order to answer questions which were not usually envisioned at the beginning of the process. This approach–creating data systems grounded in future capacity rather than limiting them to current capability–has allowed us to use data to truly support and maintain innovative programs and interorganizational linkages.

PLANNING AND ASSESSMENT PHASE

The initial task is to assess the agency's procedures and needs. This assessment is conducted during a series of in-depth interviews with directors and staff of the various programs which are going to be evaluated by our team (and tracked by the DBMS). In these interviews and discussions we focus on: (1) what are the mandated reporting needs of each program; (2) what other reports and lists of information should be made available to each program in order to facilitate program operations; (3a) what information is currently being collected by each program from new as well as currently enrolled clients, and (3b) what forms are used to collect this information and at what point are these forms filled out; (4) of the information that is currently being collected, what is the level of confidentiality required (or mandated) for various items; (5) how many different clients does each program serve each year and how many individual transactions or visits take place each year in serving this client base; (6) what are the sources from which clients are referred to each program (both intra-agency referrals and referrals by outside agencies) and what information/paperwork accompanies each type of referral; and (7) on an agency-wide basis, what are the patterns of flow of information and of paperwork? Which forms are duplicated and distributed to other programs, and which forms are kept strictly within a client's program file and not shared with other programs? What duplication exists in collecting, recording and summarizing information?

One of the inevitable initial byproducts of installing and using a data management system is the elimination of a significant amount of duplication of effort in data collection, accompanied by a standardization of many of the forms. While this process is in part a structural or logistical one, it is simultaneously a program-development process. Recognizing duplication in services and creating standardization in client-contact forms designed to capture key program information can often lead to discussions and movement toward program reorganization and staff development training.

While the clinical staff at a CBO treats patients individually and accumulates a wealth of experiential data, the social science approach to data management enables one to analyze current practices and project future needs. In each site we have found that as aggregated data were presented to–and analyzed by–the staff, the databases and report suite had to be modified a number of times. This type of participation in the production of data systems has the additional value of investing community-level staff in the data they collect for the program, and in analysis of program data.

A MODERATE SIZE COMMUNITY BASED ORGANIZATION–DSFHS

At Dominican Sisters Family Health Service[2] we initially focused on the walk-in clinic, their largest client group. Every day, DSFHS dedicated two staff members to serve clients who literally "walk-in" to their store-front offices, with needs ranging from food and shelter to immigration to HIV. A 'chart' (single record) for the first individual in a household who contacted the agency was set up containing information about that individual, the household, and the other members of the household. Each visit to the walk-in clinic was tracked, as were referrals to other services within and outside the agency. Separately, for 100 individuals covered by a Ryan White Title II grant, gross monthly data on the number of visits by each type of service provider were accumulated.

From the data in both of these databases we were able to draw profiles of the types of households being served, the range of needs of these different types of households, and how these needs change over time as the disease and family status change. Some subsequent modifications of the data collection instruments involved obtaining more household financial information (to assist in preparation of tax returns), expanding the data collected relating to risk status of clients who had been referred to the agency's Outreach programs, and more detailed tracking of outcomes. Even from these very limited data, we were able to begin to get answers to questions such as: (a) Where do clients live and how does that affect services? (b) Who refers clients and what are the implications? (c) Why do so few clients seek services for family members? (d) Why do most clients reject the offer of volunteer support? (e) What does the unit of service "short-term intervention" encompass? (f) How can we demonstrate that the program is helping clients to access entitlements? (g) What do we know about the non-compliant client; e.g., are drug users really not engageable? (h) How can ethnicity be captured in order to understand the differing needs of clients with diverse Hispanic backgrounds (the largest client group)? (i) How is this program a strategic site for health and mental health services and early intervention research?

We soon realized that the primary demographic database should not be 'client-based,' but that since DSFHS was a 'family health service,' the family's demographic profile (family ID#, name of primary householder, address, type of residence, phone, number in household, etc.) should serve as the primary database. Linked to the family database was a database of individuals which contained each individual's demographic profile (individual ID#, name, date of birth, gender, ethnicity, country of origin, relationship to the primary householder, Social Security number, Medicaid and Medicare number). We structured the ID#'s so that the family ID# was embedded within the individual ID#. Thus, even though all records of visits and services and enrollments in DSFHS programs were identified by the ID# of the individual participant, we were able to analyze the utilization of services both by each individual and by each family.

In addition to the two demographic databases, there were four databases to record activities. In the Walk-in Visit database, each record identifies the date, type of visit, the reason(s) for the visit, a narrative of the activity during, and outcome of the visit, and any referrals made as a result of the visit. These were the fields in the original form of the Visit database. However, over the years a number of other fields were added; the most important were: (a) several different versions of a detailed risk assessment, profile and risk score which were developed and modified as HIV/AIDS knowledge and approaches to prevention evolved, (b) an encoded assessment of the client's HIV knowledge and HIV status. The Program database was designed for recording each individual's enrollment in the variety of DSFHS programs (Social Work, Case Management, Therapy, Nursing, etc.) The Timesheet database was designed for recording all client-related activities within the DSFHS programs. The HIV Counseling and Testing Data Base was designed to track referrals to HIV testing and results (as reported by the clients).

A variety of reports was generated on a regular schedule (and on an ad-hoc basis when special analyses were required) and distributed to administration and staff members. The reports were used both to look at how and what the agency was doing (and how well), and as the basis for instituting changes in order to improve all aspects of operations. Here are several examples of special analyses which resulted in critical changes in agency procedures: First, over the years the ethnic makeup of the agency's catchment area in the South Bronx changed as successive waves of legal (and undocumented) immigrants found their way to DSFHS. The differing age distribution, family composition, and level of need of these groups led to changes in the spectrum of problems which had to be addressed, and in the agency's staff time allocations.

Second, as the AIDS epidemic worked its way through the community, the agency was serving more households with a 'missing generation.' Advances in drug therapy for AIDS led to an increase in the number of long-term survivors. The number of households requiring supportive services for the survivors and for the other affected household members increased, and the service needs of these households changed.

Third, the reporting requirements for the Ryan-White Title IV grant which supports much of the AIDS-related work of the agency has changed many times over the several renewal cycles of the grant (definitions of services and criteria for including a client or a service were the most frequent changes); the special reports which were needed each year for the annual reports were modified each time to match the data analyses to the new report requirements and formats.

Fourth, the agency has frequently done outreach by going to specific housing projects. We were able to supply detailed lists (by building, floor and apartment) of everyone who was known to the agency in each building allowing for very well-targeted outreach. And fifth, the agency is able to track the experiences, services and health status of families/individuals over time and use this to define outcomes and measures of success.

The DSFHS approach to CQI includes regular client record review and sustained staff development. Staff and supervisors "change their practice" and "practice change" and have been able to respond innovatively and progressively to emerging issues. The approach includes quantitative and qualitative measures to evaluate: (1) who is being reached, (2) where they are being reached, and (3) with what outcome; these methods are then modified based on this continuous feedback.The centralized database system allows DSFHS to track all agency contacts with individuals and households, e.g., case management services, psychosocial counseling services, client advocacy and Walk-In services.

A DESIGNATED AIDS CENTER–
MOUNT SINAI'S JACK MARTIN FUND CLINIC

The needs of Mount Sinai's Jack Martin Fund Clinic (JMFC) were extremely different from those of the CBO described above. The staff of the JMFC (physicians, nurses, and social workers) cared for a changing client base with an average of about 1,800 'active' cases. The database system contained no medical information and was used primarily by JMFC administration for tracking, and for internal and hospital-wide reporting. In addition to generating a group of monthly reports concerning clinic activity, productivity and physician rosters, the system was used to analyze trends in activity and to help project future needs.

The DBMS was based on three data files (Patient Demographics, Clinic Visits, and Admissions) supported by look-up databases for many fields where uniform terminology simplified analysis and reporting. The data were entered daily and audit reports were run monthly, both to verify the accuracy of the data entry and to extract data for updating several calculated fields in the Patient database. In addition to traditional demographic information, the Patient database contained date of first clinic visit and first hospital admission, JMFC physician, nurse and Social Worker team caring for the patient, date of last quality assurance review of the patient's chart by the external auditing agency and 'current' and 'final' status of the client.

The following example will demonstrate how our procedure of linking both clinic visits and hospital admissions allowed us to answer a critical clinical question and to then improve an important aspect of patient care. Each hospitalized AIDS patient is given a JMFC clinic appointment on discharge. However, JMFC clinicians knew that many inpatients did not keep those appointments but had no track of these patients.

A special report was prepared from the Admission and Visit databases for all inpatients discharged within the past 6 months. The report showed the patient's admission and discharges dates, and all clinic visits scheduled during the subsequent 6 month period, together with the outcome of each scheduled visit. We were then able to identify all of those inpatients who had not been to the JMFC following discharge. The list of those patients, sorted by Social Worker, was given to the Social Workers for follow-up. Such follow-up requires the geometry of care to extend between inpatient and outpatient settings and medical center and community-based care. Having the data infrastructure to do such follow-up on a sustained basis with support of linked databases is necessary, but not sufficient to ensure that the CQI system will be operationalized and sustained. The clinic relinquished its ability to analyze its local date on a real time basis because of financial and organizational constraints. The architecture of the system is the basis for an offshoot of this program, Health Bridge Plus which extends the geometry of care so as to support retention of the patient post discharge to include the inpatient and clinic setting data with community-based client based prevention data.

DELIVERING HOSPITAL-BASED CARE TO SRO RESIDENTS– HEALTH BRIDGE

In designing the data collection system which is used both in day-to-day operations and in continuous review and evaluation, we have successfully fused components of the CQI systems used in the DSFHS and JMFC programs. Even though the number of clients is much smaller than in either of those programs (a daily average of 120 active cases) and the staff (2 clinicians, 3 case managers, data manager and part-time data entry clerk, and evaluation consultant) the data collected, used, and analyzed is much more detailed than in those programs.

All Health Bridge clients are housed in Single Room Occupancy (SRO) residences located in the Upper West Side of Manhattan (a 15 minute walk or a single-fare bus ride from Mount Sinai). Many of the clients support themselves by temporary work, panhandling, dealing in various drugs (legal and illegal) and prostitution. All clients have an HIV/AIDS diagnosis, most have a long history of substance abuse.

Virtually all HB clients had no real connection to any aspect of the healthcare system. When first encountered, many of the clients were enrolled in Medicare (almost all are eligible for enrollment) and received sporadic, fragmented medical care by visiting one of many hospital Emergency Rooms when they felt 'really bad.'

Health Bridge was started by volunteers involved in a needle-exchange program who, as part of their 'prevention' approach to the spread of HIV/AIDS, wanted to connect needle-exchange clients to health care by providing it to them in a home-visiting program (London et al., 1998). They found a critical mass of clients by initially focusing on three SRO's and going from room to room and offering care. One of the initial sign-up programs involved offering flu vaccine.

After several months of operating with volunteer staff only, a grant was obtained under the Ryan White Title I program; this has been the sole source of funding for the program for the past six years. The reporting requirements of the Ryan White program necessitated keeping computerized records instead of an informal hand written record of each day's visits to the SRO's.

Since the hospital-based component of the medical care was to be provided by the JMFC at Mount Sinai, the obvious (and least expensive) method of collecting data was to adapt the JMFC DBMS (which had been in use at the JMFC for several years) to the needs of Health Bridge. The most important system modification which had to be made involved restructuring and expanding the Visit database to record all types of activities involved in a visit to a client in the SRO room, in addition to recording each hospital appointment scheduled.

Each action of a staff member (visit to client in SRO room, hospital visit, care coordination, telephone call, visit with no response, etc.) is recorded on a form (which has been modified many times to accommodate changing Ryan-White reporting requirements). All forms are entered in the DBMS within 3 days and a suite of reports is generated each Monday and Wednesday (to match the schedule of the Health Bridge

clinical conference held each of those mornings). At the clinical conferences, each staff member reports important changes in health status of
active clients, reviews each new client registered since the prior meeting, who should be reactivated or inactivated, etc. During the conference the reports are reviewed to plan each day's activities and to assign
responsibility for each task identified.

The suite of reports is as follows:

1. All future MSMC appointments (sorted by date and time of day).
   In addition to patient's name, the report indicates whether an escort or ambulance is needed to get to the clinic. This report is used
   by staff to plan each day's activities. (There are usually 100-120
   open appointments.)
2. All future MSMC appointments sorted by client and by date and
   time (the information is the same as in report 1, but arranging it by
   patient allows for a quick review of whether any medical service
   is missing, or the appointment schedule is too burdensome.
3. All active patients in alphabetical order showing residence, telephone number, Date of birth, Medicare number and nickname.
4. All active clients sorted by residence (same data as in report 3).
   This is the list which is used by staff when they make their rounds
   in each SRO. It is arranged so that the SRO residents are listed by
   floor and room, starting at the highest floor (this allows staff to
   take the elevator to the top floor, work their way door to door
   along each hallway, then walk down the stairs to the next floor.
5. All hospitalized clients, showing name, ward and admission date.
6. The outcome (completed, missed, cancelled, rescheduled) of each
   clinic appointment during the prior week. (This is used to see what
   appointments have to be rescheduled and which clients might
   need some extra attention, such as being escorted to appointments.) (This report is only printed for the Monday clinical conference.)

In addition to this suite of operating reports, summary reports were
prepared monthly for filling out the Ryan White reports and for entering
the data into the Uniform Reporting System (URS) which was instituted
during the fourth year of the project.

One of the most unique (and useful) reports we were able to generate
was a complete chronological list of all contacts and appointments
(completed and/or missed) for each client. This report enabled us to
demonstrate how much effort, and how many steps, were often required

in order to 'connect' with a client, convince the client to allow a Health Bridge clinician to examine him in his room, and then eventually link the client with a JMFC clinician (and any necessary specialty clinics).

Once the initial medical connection with a client was established by Health Bridge staff, most clients were found to have a substantial number of medical, social, and family problems in addition to AIDS. Specialty services provided directly by the JMFC include psychiatry, dermatology, ophthalmology, ob/gyn, neurology, renal and adherence counseling. A major benefit (to the clients and to the medical care system) occurs when instead of going to an Emergency Room, many HB clients took advantage of the Urgent Care walk-in clinic at the JMFC where they can be seen immediately by a nurse-practitioner (who often already knows the client and has immediate access to the client's clinical charts and history).

Virtually all Health Bridge clients were not in medical care when HB first encountered them (Indyk, London, Tackley, Wennberg, & Heller, 1998). All of them had been diagnosed with AIDS (often during incarceration) and all had virtually no confidence or trust in the medical care system. Many of the clients continued to engage in a variety of unsafe sexual practices, many use a variety of illegal substances, and go in and out of rehab programs. Most were perceived by the medical establishment (generally when they were brought to a hospital Emergency Room) as 'extremely difficult' patients.

One of the major challenges to maintaining continuity of care for these clients is the 'revolving door' aspect of their housing. Often, when a client is hospitalized or incarcerated for an extended period, his room is closed and then given to someone else. HB staff make daily visits to all HB clients who are hospitalized and work very closely with the hospital staff in discharge planning to make certain that no one falls through the cracks and that the special needs of each HB client are addressed.

Another example of the problems associated with providing care to the HB client group can be elicited by examining the Medicaid Sequence number. Each time a client loses his Medicaid card (or it is stolen), he must get a new card. The Sequence number indicates the number of times a card has been replaced (and medical care such as clinic visits, prescription refills, etc. has had to be interrupted). In the current active group of 124 clients, 38 have a sequence number over 20 (the highest is 49).

The data system and standardized reporting routines have been refined over the years to enable the HB clinical and case management staff to provide the level of intensive and appropriate care and follow-up necessary to high retention and survival rates. Each day the full hospital census report is scanned by the staff to see if any 'inactive' HB clients are in-patients. Anyone who was at any time enrolled in HB is visited and, if appropriate, his case is reactivated. A periodic report of 'date of last contact' is used to see with whom the staff should touch base on their daily rounds of the SRO's.

Each month, a report of all JMFC appointments and hospitalizations of AIDS clients is downloaded from the MSMC data system. These reports are compared with our data to make certain that all activities of HB clients have been captured by our DBMS. The MSMC reports are also used to find any 'inactive' HB clients who continue to attend the JMFC clinic.

Health Bridge was originally developed in response to discovering that people living with HIV/AIDS in SROs were mostly not connected to care. Although it was initially believed that the Health Bridge population represented outliers in the population of HIV infected individuals, we have found that more than half of the inpatients admitted with HIV infection, on any given day, are not in care. The DBMS provided an infrastructure for connecting the dots within and between community, clinic and inpatient settings. We are increasingly applying the lessons learned in Health Bridge to clients identified in the inpatient unit who similarly require a re-engineering of the geometry of care they are receiving so as to include pathways between and across systems to support their retention in care. We are expanding the Health Bridge model to support engagement and retention from the inside out as well as from the outside in.

CONCLUSION

We have described (in a variety of settings), how our efforts to support a Continuous Quality Improvement to data capacity building using very sophisticated data collection and reporting have enabled us to assist front line providers to evaluate their efforts and outcomes (in real time) and, to enhance the care they are able to provide with limited resources. Each setting is strategically positioned to reach individuals at different points along the continuum of risk and disease and, with tools and technical assistance, to describe populations and individuals reached at these points. Advances in treatment have created a population living with HIV, mental illness, addictions and other medical co-morbidities which require medical management, health maintenance and support of patient behavior modification. Management of HIV requires complex management over time of acute, chronic and life style issues. The geometry of care should ideally have at its center, an informed patient who, with appropriate consultative support has the motivation, knowledge and ability to be aware of emerging problems, and have access to systems of treatment, support and prevention. A large percentage of individuals with HIV infection are either unaware of their status or not in any or consistent care. The locus of care shifts depending upon where an individual reaches or is reached by various systems. In the current fragmented health care system, development of a bottom-up data-management system can take advantage of existing institutional data sets as well as creatively develop its unique management system tailored to its particular needs and strengths.

REFERENCES

Indyk, D., & Indyk, L. (1995). "Filling in the Blanks: Creating and Aggregating Service Driven Data to Develop Community Profiles of Special Population." In Data Needs in an Era of Health Reform. Proceedings of the 25th Public Health Conference on Records and Statistics and the National Committee on Vital and Health Statistics 45th Anniversary Symposium, pp. 398-402.

Indyk, D., London, K., Tackley, L., Wennberg, J., & Heller, D. (1998). "Innovative model for the provision of HIV primary care to persons otherwise lost to follow-up by traditional medical delivery systems. Presented at the 12th World AIDS Conference, Geneva, July, 2, 1998. [Abstract # 42312].

London, K., Indyk, D., Clark, J., Stancliff, S., Lee, A., & Nardi, S. (1998). "Results of a clinical outreach to HIV infected individuals living in SRO hotels. Presented at the 12th World AIDS Conference, Geneva, June, 29, 1998. [Abstract # 12447].

A Community-Based Organization's Integration of HIV and Substance Abuse Treatment Services for Ex-Offenders

Danielle Strauss, MPH

SUMMARY. This paper explores the point of intersection of the substance abuse treatment and HIV services industries with the criminal justice system. Section I reviews the literature and "best practices" that have integrated substance abuse treatment and HIV care and prevention services for ex-offenders and which informed the development of a community-based organization's initiative, the VIP STRIVE Project. Section II presents a brief history of VIP in the context of its ability to adapt to its environment and to the changing needs of its target population,

---

Danielle Strauss, MPH, is affiliated with the Hunter College School of Social Work, City University of New York.

For their time and thoughtful contributions and perspectives, the author thanks Sandra Ruiz Butter, President of VIP Community Services; Dr. John Carway, Vice President of Program Services for VIP Community Services; Warren Morrisett, Vice President for Health Services for VIP Community Services; Damien Cabezas, Assistant Vice President for Program Services and; Alma Candelas, Director of the Bureau of Special Populations for the New York State Department of Health, AIDS Institute.

This paper was written for a class in Hunter College's PhD program for Social Welfare. It is based on an extensive review of the literature as well as the author's personal experience as Program Director for HIV Prevention for VIP Community Services. Interviews with key figures from VIP and NYS-based funding institutions were conducted in order to thoroughly develop and present the main concepts of this paper.

[Haworth co-indexing entry note]: "A Community-Based Organization's Integration of HIV and Substance Abuse Treatment Services for Ex-Offenders." Strauss, Danielle. Co-published simultaneously in *Social Work in Health Care* (The Haworth Press, Inc.) Vol. 42, No. 3/4, 2006, pp. 61-76; and: *The Geometry of Care: Linking Resources, Research, and Community to Reduce Degrees of Separation Between HIV Treatment and Prevention* (ed: Debbie Indyk) The Haworth Press, Inc., 2006, pp. 61-76. Single or multiple copies of this article are available for a fee from The Haworth Document Delivery Service [1-800-HAWORTH, 9:00 a.m. - 5:00 p.m. (EST). E-mail address: docdelivery@haworthpress.com].

Available online at http://www.haworthpress.com/web/SWHC
doi:10.1300/J010v42n03_05

with specific reference to the development of HIV and substance abuse treatment services for members of the criminal justice population. The concluding section brings the two previous sections together by explaining how the VIP STRIVE Project can assist VIP in enhancing its capacity to integrate its substance abuse treatment and HIV services in order to improve services for this target population. *[Article copies available for a fee from The Haworth Document Delivery Service: 1-800-HAWORTH. E-mail address: <docdelivery@haworthpress.com> Website: <http://www.HaworthPress.com> © 2006 by The Haworth Press, Inc. All rights reserved.]*

KEYWORDS. Substance abuse, harm-reduction, HIV, integration, care

Injection drug use (IDU) accounts for over one-third (36%) of all AIDS cases in the United States since the epidemic began in the early 1980s (SAMHSA, 2002). This figure includes individuals directly infected through injection drug practice, as well as those indirectly infected through sexual contact with an infected IDU or mother-to-child transmission. In fact, 57% of all AIDS cases among women have been attributed to IDU or sexual contact with an infected IDU, compared to only 31% of all male cases. In addition to injection drug use, alcohol and cocaine have been associated with an increased risk for HIV infection (Samet, Mulvey, Zaremba & Plough, 1999).

The role of IV drug use in HIV infection is particularly salient in communities of color. According to the *Health Emergency 2003* report, among those who inject drugs, African Americans are 5 times more likely and Latinos are 1 1/2 times more likely as whites to get AIDS (Day, 2002). SAMHSA (2002) further reported that in 2000, 26% of all IDU-related AIDS cases were among African Americans and 31% were among Hispanics, compared to only 19% among whites.

Complicating the relationship between substance use and HIV infection is the disproportionate impact that the "War on Drugs" has had on communities of color (Mauer, 2003). According to the Bureau of Justice Statistics (Bureau of Justice, 2003 [Nov 16]), African Americans are five times more likely to be incarcerated than whites and twice as likely to be imprisoned as Latinos. In fact, one in three African American males is expected to go to prison in his lifetime, as compared to one in six Hispanic males and one in 17 white males (Bonczar, 2003). Moreover, while only 11% of the nation's drug users are black, African Americans constitute almost 37% of those arrested for drug violations

(SAMHSA, 1997), over 47% of those in federal prisons for drug violations (Bureau of Justice Statistics [BJS]1997), and almost 60% of those in state prisons for drug felonies (BJS, 1997a).

Not surprisingly, HIV/AIDS is highly prevalent among members of the incarcerated population, primarily due to its interrelationship with substance abuse. According to the Bureau of Justice Statistics, 2% of prison inmates were known to be HIV-positive in 2000. However, when the data was broken down by State, 8.5% of New York's prison inmates were HIV-infected, which was nearly a quarter of all inmates known to be HIV positive in 2000, and the largest proportion for the country (Maruschak, 2002). Furthermore, the rate of confirmed AIDS cases was four times higher for prison inmates than the general population (Maruschak, 2002).

Finally, compounding this relationship between substance use, incarceration, and HIV infection is the additional problem of recidivism within the criminal justice system. The Bureau of Justice Statistics indicates that about 20% of criminal offenders admitted to prison in 1998 on drug charges were on parole at the time of arrest and 44% were on probation. In addition, 80% of drug-offenders had a prior offense or sentence on record and over half had served three or more sentences prior to 1998 (Wilson, 2000). A meta-analysis of the role of substance abuse factors in predicting recidivism suggested that drug or alcohol abuse was in fact the strongest predictor for recidivism (Dowden & Brown, 2002). Interestingly, a prior drug charge did not prove to be a significant predictor for recidivism (Dowden & Brown, 2002), indicating that the problem had more to do with ongoing substance abuse rather than a history of incarceration.

These intersecting issues–substance use, incarceration, and recidivism–represent a case example of the new geometry of care necessary to effectively treat HIV-positive individuals and prevent the spread of new infections (Rier & Indyk, this volume). This article outlines the evolution of the integration of HIV and re-entry services into VIP's portfolio of programs in response to both funding opportunities and community needs. The SAMHSA-funded initiative, STRIVE (Substance Abuse Treatment Referrals through InnoVative Education and Support), which aims to reach out to ex-offenders from the criminal justice system and prepare them for HIV care and substance abuse treatment services in the community, was elaborated through this iterative process.

LITERATURE REVIEW AND BEST PRACTICES

Substance Abuse Treatment and HIV/AIDS

In 2001, the Centers for Disease Control and Prevention (CDC) commissioned the Academy for Educational Development (AED) to conduct a review of several studies that looked at the integration of HIV services with substance abuse treatment programs, primarily methadone maintenance programs. Results indicated that treatment programs could have a dramatic effect on HIV transmission among injection drug users, reducing their risk by 40-60% (CDC, 2002). The majority of these programs offered HIV counseling/testing onsite. However, several others added other HIV prevention components, including incorporating HIV prevention messages into basic substance abuse treatment education and counseling, using HIV outreach strategies for reaching out-of-treatment IDUs and linking them to treatment programs, encouraging syringe exchange, and using family counseling to work with patient's sexual partners and children (CDC, 2002).

Findings from a study looking at the effect of entering drug treatment as a means for reducing drug use and HIV-related risk behavior supported the idea that entry into drug treatment substantially reduced drug use among out-of-treatment users and also reduced HIV-related risk behavior (Hoffman, Klein, Clark, & Boyd, 1998). However, the study found that there was a high rate of relapse among the participants post-treatment (Hoffman et al., 1998).

Although challenging to evaluate, HIV outreach programs are believed to be effective at reaching out-of-treatment drug users and reducing their risk of HIV transmission, while developing their readiness for drug treatment and referring them into drug treatment when they are ready (Booth & Koester, 1996, CDC, 2004, Greenberg & Neumann, 1998).

Looking at readiness for drug treatment as a predictor for success in treatment, Czuchry and Dansereau (2003) found that drug users with higher levels of readiness demonstrated a greater involvement in the treatment program and therefore a greater likelihood of success. The authors found this to be particularly true for ex-offenders and probationers. Similarly, Neff and Zule (2002) sought to understand variations in substance abuse treatment use by focusing on the following factors that might predict readiness for treatment: "perceived problem severity," "perceived need for formal treatment," "motivation for treatment," and "negative attitudes toward treatment." The authors found that "motivation to quit" was the only significant predictor for use of all types of drug treatment, while "perceived need for treatment" plus "motivation to quit" were significant predictors for use or attempted use (Neff & Zule, 2002). Thus, programs that address these factors prior to referring clients to treatment could assist clients in having greater success in treatment once referred.

Substance Abuse Treatment and the Criminal Justice System

The need for substance abuse treatment programs within the criminal justice system and post-discharge to prevent recidivism has been known and addressed extensively over the past decade. In 1998, 72.8% of all jails provided some form of substance abuse treatment for their inmates, including detoxification, counseling, residential treatment, basic education programs, and/or self-help programs such as Narcotics Anonymous (N.A.) or Alcoholics Anonymous (A.A.) (Wilson, 2000). However, only 12% of these jails provided all types of treatment programs, offering inmates a full-range of treatment options and intensities, and about 22% offered only the self-help programs (which is the least intensive and the least costly) (Wilson, 2000).

While more than half of all jail inmates convicted on drug-related charges reported participation in some form of drug treatment program during their incarceration, only about one fourth of all state and federal prison inmates reported the same (BIJ, 2003a). Similarly, only slightly more than one-third of all adults placed on probation with a suspended sentence on the condition that they received substance abuse treatment, reported having received such treatment (BIJ, 2003a).

However, within the past decade, the criminal justice system has experimented with another, possibly more effective strategy for mandating offenders to drug treatment. This strategy is called "Alternatives to Incarceration" or "Drug Court." Drug court judges sentence drug offenders to drug treatment instead of prison or jail. The State Sentencing and Corrections Program of the Vera Institute of Justice issued a report in 2000 presenting data on the success of such programs. This report stated that nearly every published evaluation of drug court concluded that graduates of the program were less likely to return to prison or jail than non-graduates (Fluellen & Trone, 2000). It further cited two specific studies, one from the King County Drug Court in Washington State and the other from the Okaloosa and Escambia Drug Courts in Florida that had outcome data demonstrating the success of their programs. The King County Drug Court study found that its graduates were three times less likely to be charged with a new crime one year after completing treatment, as compared to those who dropped out of the program or were never enrolled (Fluellen & Trone 2000). Similarly, in Okaloosa, 26% of the graduates of the program were rearrested 30 months post-discharge, as compared to 63% of those who dropped out. In Escambia, almost half of the graduates were rearrested, as compared to more than three-fourths (86%) of those who did not complete the program (ibid). According to the authors of this report, the lessons from these studies included the need for drug court programs to strengthen their capacity to retain offenders in their treatment programs, so that they don't drop out, get the full benefit of treatment, and avoid relapse and recidivism in the future (Fluellen & Trone 2000).

Overcoming drug abuse is often a lifetime struggle. While the criminal justice system offers some drug treatment programs during incarceration, there is not enough assistance and support for drug offenders after they are discharged or complete mandated treatment programs. Recognizing that relapse is normal and part of the recovery process, inmates linked to longer-term and community-based drug treatment programs post-discharge may have greater success in maintaining sobriety after they have reentered the community, and therefore may be better prepared for a new life outside of prison or jail. Without such support, it should be no surprise that most return to drugs and are at some point rearrested and reconvicted, further disrupting their lives, their relationships with their families and community, and their ability to contribute positively to society.

HIV/AIDS and the Criminal Justice System

Like the provision of drug treatment in prison and jails, the United States Criminal Justice System offers programs related to HIV care and prevention for inmates. Such programs include HIV counseling/testing and case management and medical treatment for those prisoners infected with HIV. In a study conducted in Seattle, Washington, a group of HIV positive offenders were compared to a similar group of HIV negative offenders. The study tracked both groups after discharge. Within three months of discharge, 50% of both groups were rearrested. However, during the following three to six months, the HIV positive individuals were significantly more likely to be rearrested (Harris, Rafii, Tonge & Uldall, 2002). The authors concluded by explaining the possible relationship between being HIV positive and recidivism. They attributed the re-arrest to ongoing drug use, but they also considered the relationship between commercial sex work (which is illegal) and HIV, as well as the fact that HIV-infected individuals might seek incarceration to obtain medical treatment that they were denied outside of prison (Harris et al., 2002).

In recognition of this need to link HIV-infected inmates to medical treatment programs post-discharge, the Centers for Disease Control and Prevention (CDC) and Health Resources Services Administration (HRSA) funded several demonstration projects in 1999, to identify successful strategies and best practices. The premise behind these projects was that the criminal justice system was in a good position to screen inmates for HIV through the provision of onsite HIV counseling/testing services, educate them about HIV prevention, and provide medical treatment for those who tested positive (Potter, 2003). During discharge planning, caseworkers referred the HIV-infected inmates to local community-based organizations (CBOs) funded by the Ryan White Care Act, for HIV primary care and follow up post-discharge. These Ryan White Care programs were also funded by HRSA, which reinforced the funding agency's ability to strengthen the linkages. The inmates were assigned a case manager from the CBO, who was responsible for following up on the individuals after they were discharged and assisting them with maintaining their medication regimens and keeping medical appointments (Potter, 2003). Thus, the aim was to have a smooth transition from the prison or jail setting back into the community, at least with regard to their healthcare.

Two factors were identified as requisites for the success of these programs. One was that the bureaucratic structures of both the criminal justice and public health systems facilitated the clear delineation of roles, responsibilities and accountability among the staff members involved in the linkage. The other factor was that correctional facilities and health departments that had prior experience working with each other were deemed more successful (Potter, 2003). However, several barriers were also identified, including the high turnover of jail inmate populations, which compromised the continuity of care, as well as the difference in each system's mission, which made it difficult for many staff members from both sides to understand each other and work together. Despite these barriers, the author stated that such collaborations were possible and crucial for those communities disproportionately affected by crime and disease (Potter, 2003). Unfortunately, as with substance abuse treatment, successful collaborations between the criminal justice system and HIV-related community-based treatment programs are rare.

SYSTEM LEVEL GEOMETRY:
THE CONFLUENCE OF SUBSTANCE ABUSE,
HIV AND INCARCERATION

Effective treatment and prevention services for both HIV and Substance Abuse require the development of a continuum of these services which match appropriate levels of need and readiness of individuals to engage in these services. The challenge presented by the intersection of substance use, HIV, and the criminal justice system is that it requires the creation and maintenance of multiple programmatic linkages that (simultaneously) support primary, secondary and tertiary prevention of HIV, substance misuse and recidivism. The integration of these services requires the development of a web of internal and external linkages which support multiple entry points to prevention and treatment. Incarcerated individuals with HIV disease and addictions need support upon re-entry into community not only with medication management, but also with an array of daily challenges that put them at further risk for relapse and recidivism.

In 1999, SAMHSA (the Substance Abuse Mental Health Services Administration), initiated the HIV outreach grants initiative, with funding from the Minority AIDS Task Force (formally known as the Congressional Black Caucus) (SAMHSA, 2002). The purpose of this funding was to reduce drug-using behavior and encourage treatment by successfully employing outreach techniques to reach this high-risk population (SAMHSA, 2004). VIP Community Services was among the first group of CBOs to receive this funding. A Bronx based multi-service substance abuse treatment agency with an array of HIV care and prevention services, VIP was at the "vanguard" of treatment and prevention services for this population (c.f. Rier & Indyk, this volume) and was in a strategic position to pioneer these linkages.

The VIP STRIVE Project

The VIP STRIVE Project was designed to address both the substance abuse and HIV prevention and treatment needs of its target population. The program utilizes outreach and in-reach as tools through which to engage individuals in low-threshold, harm reduction services that support HIV prevention. But, unlike earlier HIV outreach programs, it doesn't market Counseling and Testing as its only product. Since individuals are at different stages of readiness to seek and accept substance abuse, mental health, and/or HIV medical treatment, the program tailors its outreach to support entry, engagement and retention in care. Client-centered 'outreach and engagement' requires the development of linkages within and between HIV, substance use, and mental health systems of care and prevention, which must be tapped to support the emerging needs of clients.

The project engages substance users through an array of low- to medium-threshold services, in order to assist them in developing a readiness for treatment prior to being referred into formal treatment programs. Low-threshold services refer to outreach and other types of HIV risk reduction activities that require very little effort on the part of the client or community member. The CDC (1998) defines such activities as those that "employ peers or paraprofessionals to reach large numbers of people with less time-intensive, staff-intensive risk reduction strategies."

This is in contrast to medium-threshold services such as prevention case management. According to the CDC (1998), prevention case management is an individual-level HIV prevention intervention characterized by formal enrollment of clients into ongoing services for approximately 4-6 months, the development of a formal relationship between a prevention case manager and a client, with in-depth, on-going risk reduction counseling that addresses behavioral change objectives specific to the needs of that one particular client. In addition to prevention case management, the VIP STRIVE Project offers other medium-threshold services, including curriculum-based behavior-change workshops (i.e., Anger Management, Stress Management, Relapse Prevention, Parenting Skills, etc.) and ongoing support groups for substance users living with HIV or affected in some other way.

The ultimate goal of the project is to outreach and engage members of this target population in these medium-threshold services, and to keep them engaged for a period of at least 6 months, in order to help develop their readiness for longer-term and higher-threshold services prior to being referred. Higher-threshold services refer to those programs that last for over 6 months, require life-long maintenance skills, and have sustained impact on the clients' lives. These services include, but are not limited to, substance abuse treatment, HIV medical treatment, and mental health treatment. Other examples of higher-threshold programs include vocational counseling and training and housing assistance.

VIP's System Level Changes Made in Response to a Changing Environment

The epidemic spread of HIV in the late 1980s profoundly, though belatedly, changed the nature of drug treatment services in New York City. It was an epidemic that spread so fast and targeted such specifically vulnerable populations that both the health care and drug treatment systems are still reeling from the impact, two decades later.

The first target population for HIV/AIDS services was Gay men. But by 1987, the New York State Department of Health, AIDS Institute, began seeing a change in the epidemic, with Injection Drug Users (IDUs) surpassing Men who have Sex with Men (MSM) in numbers of new AIDS cases per year. With funding from the CDC, the AIDS Institute joined forces with the Department of Substance Abuse Services (DSAS–later to merge with the Department of Alcohol Services, to form the Office of Alcohol and Substance Abuse Services or OASAS). This joint venture led to the initiation of the Counseling, Testing, Referral, and Partner Notification (CTRPN) Initiative in 1989. This initiative located HIV counseling/testing sites within already established substance abuse treatment programs identified by OASAS, which were primarily methadone maintenance programs at that time. By 1990, the initiative expanded to include HIV primary care services.

The purpose of this initiative was to reach substance users in treatment who were possibly infected with HIV and get them tested and into care. Thus, substance abuse treatment acted as an entry point for HIV services. VIP received this initial funding for HIV counseling/testing in 1991, and then expanded to include primary care in 1992.

At this time, the substance abuse treatment industry and most substance abuse treatment providers were in a state of crisis. Clients were getting sick and dying at epidemic rates. In addition, being an industry notorious for its use of paraprofessionals, specifically former substance users, many staff members who were infected in the 1980s were dying as well. The substance abuse treatment programs felt like they had to do something, but they had no idea what to do. Prior to HIV, the substance abuse treatment industry focused on the clients' substance abuse problem, and little attention was given to other issues or problems in their clients' lives. Furthermore, drug treatment programs tended to be isolated from health care settings who at that time were not ready, willing or equipped to work with individuals actively using substances. HIV forced substance abuse providers to look at their clients as human beings, recognize the need to address their health problems in addition to their substance abuse problem, and take a more holistic approach to treatment.

VIP was no exception. Although already open to being a multi-modality site, the provision of health services, specifically HIV services, for clients in treatment, and later for the community, introduced concepts to VIP such as harm reduction, client-centeredness, and the integration of services. VIP's HIV services broadened VIP's thinking as well as forced the agency to get involved with other agencies in the community to develop a referral network and collaboration.

What started as a small HIV counseling/testing and primary care program in 1992, with a budget of approximately $200,000, grew into a full-fledged Health Services Department that offers full primary care services, HIV prevention and enhanced services specifically for women. By 2003, VIP's Health Services Department's budget was over $2 million, with funding from local, state and federal levels as well as Medicaid.

However, HIV treatment advances forced changes in the HIV/AIDS industry over the course of the decade, opening new doors for VIP, while threatening to close some old ones. The early 90s were times of urgency and panic. People were dying and there was no magic bullet for treatment or prevention. The stigma of AIDS impacted individuals living with AIDS as well as those working with the infected. Many of the programs that were funded in those early years couldn't even fill positions with clinicians. In recognition of the immensity of the problem and the lack of experience on the part of substance abuse treatment providers in dealing with health issues, the AIDS Institute included vast amounts of staff training, support for community-based networks, and technical assistance in its initial funding cycle.

A major visionary and leader in the field, Dr. Nick Rango, Medical Director of the AIDS Institute at that time, further appreciated the treatment agencies' need for infrastructure development in order to adapt to the requirements for the provision of HIV services, and made available to them opportunities for additional funding through the Multi-Service Agency (MSA) grants. With MSA money, VIP was able to develop and expand its technological capacity to be able to capture client-level data, so that today, VIP has one of the most sophisticated information technology systems in the Bronx.

By the mid-90s, however, the discovery of HIV medications offered in combination, known as the triple cocktail or HAART therapy, transformed HIV from a fatal disease to a chronic illness. As a result of this technological breakthrough in AIDS research, the cost of HIV medications skyrocketed at the same moment in time when managed care and other cost efficiency concepts were taking hold and threatening agency funding. The AIDS Institute was no longer able to sustain the intensive amount of funding and technical assistance that it provided during the early 1990s. Furthermore, as competition for funding increased, all of the networks of providers that were established during the early 90s felt threatened as agencies became more reluctant to collaborate, share experiences and lessons learned, and cross refer, for fear of losing clients and funding to other agencies.

In an effort to stay ahead of the curve and be prepared for possible cutbacks to Medicaid and grant funding, VIP's Board of Directors initiated a process to reexamine its goals and objectives and future plans during a strategic planning meeting in 1997. An outcome of this meeting was a decision to restructure the agency, which involved a change in Board Chair, changes in job titles from the more non-profit sounding Executive Director and Assistant Executive Director, to the more corporate sounding President and Vice-President, and to revise the agency's mission statement to a more generic one that could appeal to any potential funder. This process was initiated in response to the growing expectation that non-profits function more like businesses and focus more on efficiency and cost-effective practices.

Thus, by the late 90s, VIP's primary care services had expanded to include services to the community at large, as a result of an effort to expand medical services beyond HIV in case funding for HIV care ever disappeared. Meanwhile, now that the treatment for HIV was stabilized, funders were focusing less on funding care programs and more on prevention. VIP received its first prevention grant from the New York City Department of Health in March 1997 and a second one from the CDC in October 1997. This CDC grant was the first federally funded program for VIP, which lead to greater visibility for the agency and the beginnings of national recognition. In 1999, VIP received two substantial HIV prevention grants from SAMHSA-CSAT. One was specifically to provide at-risk women with enhanced treatment, which led to the development of VIP's Women's Center, a safe place and drop-in center for active drug using women as well as those in treatment. The other SAMHSA grant (referred to in the Introduction) was to develop HIV outreach and prevention services as an entry point into substance abuse treatment.

Thus, by this point in the epidemic, substance abuse treatment programs were no longer the entry point for HIV, but rather the HIV outreach and prevention services, being relatively low-threshold and based on harm reduction principles, acted as entry points for entry into substance abuse treatment. This program funded by SAMHSA established the Prevention Unit within VIP as its own entity and launched VIP, an agency with roots in substance abuse treatment, into the realm of outreach and harm reduction for active drug users.

By embracing the notion of "meeting the clients where they are at" and assisting them in reducing their risk, as opposed to practicing abstinence, the Women's Center and Prevention Unit practiced and demonstrated outcomes of client-centered treatment. This occurred at the same time that the agency's senior management became interested in the concept of the client-centered approach. Management saw this as a welcome alternative to the more traditional substance abuse treatment philosophy that viewed substance abuse as a disease and substance abusers as powerless, leaving all the power in the hands of the treatment provider, only to blame the client when the treatment failed. As a result, VIP has embraced the concept of the client-centered approach on an agency level, incorporated the concept into its newly revised mission statement and is in the process of providing all clinical staff with extensive training and supervision on this new model and philosophy towards drug treatment and the substance abuse client.

While the HIV services were expanding and transforming VIP on one level, the substance abuse treatment industry was responding to yet another change in its environment, which further transformed VIP during this turbulent decade. During the mid-90s, Janet Reno, the Attorney General under President Clinton, initiated the drug court program. This program linked substance abuse treatment agencies to the criminal justice system, allowing offenders charged with drug-related crimes to be mandated into treatment as an alternative to incarceration. VIP recognized the significance of this program for the future of drug treatment and made sure the agency was at the table during the initial meetings to establish a Drug Court in the Bronx. Bronx Court selected VIP as one of five providers in the Bronx.

As a result of this linkage, VIP's client population changed from the older substance user entering treatment as a self-referral after s/he had hit bottom, to a much younger and angrier client mandated to treatment. Furthermore, an increasing number of clients started presenting with mental health issues, known as the MICA (Mentally Ill, Chemically Dependent) client. Thus services had to be adapted to meet the needs of this new and much more vulnerable and difficult-to-work-with population.

Meanwhile, the substance abuse treatment industry was further transforming itself as it became more professionalized. In 1996, OASAS established the Certification for Alcohol and Substance Abuse Counseling (CASAC). As grant funding diminished more and more substance abuse treatment programs needed to make the transition to third party reimbursement for survival. However, third parties, including Medicaid, refused to reimburse for certain services unless they were implemented by what they called "certified health professionals" (an individual with a CASAC and/or a Masters Degree in Social Work or equivalent). As a result of this change, VIP had to revise its job requirements for its Substance Abuse Counselors. Prior to the CASAC and third party restrictions, most Substance Abuse Counselors were paraprofessionals who were members of the community, who themselves were in recovery and therefore able to relate to clients, as well as were more likely to match clients racially and ethnically. Now, with the above restrictions, more staff members were being hired with CASACs and/or MSWs. Thus, VIP is accepting better academically trained personnel less likely to have the same or similar background as the clients. The impact of this change on the clients, services and outcomes of treatment remains to be seen.

CONCLUSION

While VIP's HIV care and prevention services expanded and diversified over the previous decade, in response to developments in the HIV industry as well as changes to funding, so did substance abuse treatment programs. Unfortunately, despite the early recognition of their interrelatedness during the late 80s and early 90s, it appears that the two have evolved independently of each other. What started out for VIP as a small HIV program well integrated within a much larger and more dominant substance abuse treatment agency has become two separate and equally strong departments, held together by the overarching administrative body, but not well-integrated.

The VIP STRIVE Project is therefore an opportunity for VIP to bring these two arms of the agency closer by establishing a linkage between the two departments that are, once again, essentially serving the same target population. As previously stated, the VIP STRIVE Project is designed to outreach to members of the criminal justice population and facilitate their entry into treatment by providing them with low-medium threshold HIV prevention services and developing their readiness for treatment prior to referral. VIP's substance abuse treatment modalities are now serving an increasing number of ex-offenders mandated to treatment and have developed their services to specifically meet the needs of this population. Furthermore, the treatment modalities are under more and more pressure to demonstrate positive outcomes and results. Thus, the VIP STRIVEs Project can and should assist these modalities by outreaching and working with clients prior to entering treatment, preparing them for treatment, and enhancing their treatment experience once in treatment, through the application of the client-centered and harm reduction approach. If primary prevention is deemed not a feasible economic goal, it would serve the industry well to demonstrate that the safety net in fact will lead to higher retention in treatment, lower recidivism and prove to be a cost-effective, efficacious and critical component of the care continuum in the long run.

REFERENCES

Bonczar, T.P. (2003 August). Prevalence of Imprisonment in the U.S. Population, 1974-2001. *Bureau of Justice Statistics Special Report.*

Booth, R.E. and Koester, S.K. (1996, Summer). Issues and approaches to evaluating HIV outreach interventions. *Journal on Drug Issues.* Vol. 26, Issue 3.

Bureau of Justice Statistics. (1997). Sourcebook of Criminal Justice Statistics 1996. Tables 4.10 and 6.36.

Bureau of Justice Statistics. (1997a). Prisoners in 1996. Table 13.

Bureau of Justice Statistics. (2003, November 16). Criminal Offender Statistics. Retrieved November 27, 2003 from *http://www.ojp.usdoj.gov/bjs/crimoff.htm*

Bureau of Justice Statistics. (2003). Drug Treatment Under Correctional Supervision. Retrieved December 4, 2003 from *http://www.ojp.usdoj.gov/bjs/dcf/dt.htm*

Centers for Disease Control and Prevention. (2003, Dec. 24). Community PROMISE: Peers reaching out and modeling intervention strategies for HIV/AIDS risk reduction in their community. Centers for Disease Control and Prevention, National Center for HIV, STD, and TB Prevention, Division of HIV/AIDS Prevention.

Centers for Disease Control and Prevention. (1998, January 26). HIV prevention case management–Guidance: September Centers for Disease Control and Prevention, National Center for HIV, STD, and TB Prevention, Division of HIV/AIDS Prevention.

Centers for Disease Control and Prevention. (2002, February). Linking HIV prevention services and substance abuse treatment programs. *IDU/HIV Prevention.* Produced by the Academy for Educational Development.

Czuchry, M. and Dansereau, D.F. (2003, February). Cognitive skills training: impact on drug abuse counseling and readiness for treatment. *American Journal of Drug and Alcohol Abuse.* Retrieved April 8, 2004, from http://www.findarticles.com/cf_dls/m0978/1_29/101175126/print.jhtml

Day, D. (2002). Health Emergency 2003: The Spread of Drug-Related AIDS and Hepatitis C Among African American and Latinos. Harm Reduction Coalition.

Dowden, C. and Brown, S.L. (2002). The Role of Substance Abuse Factors in Predicting Recidivism: A Meta-Analysis. *Psychology, Crime & Law,* Vol. 8, pp. 243-264.

Fluellen, R. and Trone, J. (2000). Do drug courts save jail and prison beds?: Issues in Brief. The State Sentencing and Corrections Program at the Vera Institute of Justice.

Greenberg, J.B. and Neumann, M.S. (1998). What we have learned from the AIDS evaluation of street outreach project: A summary document. Centers for Disease Control and Prevention, Atlanta, GA.

Harris, V.L., Rafii, R., Tonge, S.J., and Uldall, K.K. (2002). Rearrest: does HIV serostatus make a difference? *AIDS Care*, Vol. 14, No. 6, pp. 839-849.

Hoffman, J. A., Klein, H., Clark, D. C., and Boyd, F. T. (1998, May). The effect of entering drug treatment on involvement in HIV-related risk behaviors. (The NIDA Cooperative Agreement for AIDS Community-based Outreach/intervention Research Programs)(National Institute on Drug Abuse). *American Journal of Drug and Alcohol Abuse*. Retrieved April 8, 2004 from *http://www.findarticles. com/cf_dls/m0978/ n2_v24/20842697/print.jhtml*

Human Rights Watch. (2000). United States–Punishment and Prejudice: Racial Disparities in the War on Drugs, I. Summary and Recommendations. Retrieved Dec. 1, 2003 from *http://www.hrw.org/reports/2000/usa/Rcedrg00.htm*

Koroloffe, N.M. and Briggs, H.E. (1996). The life cycle of family advocacy organizations. *Administration in Social Work*. Vol. 20 (4).

Maruschak, L.M. (2002, October). HIV in Prisons, 2000. *Bureau of Justice Statistics Bulletin*.

Mauer, M. (2003, June 20). Comparative International Rates of Incarceration: An Examination of Causes and Trends. The Sentencing Project.

Meyer, A.L., Goes, J.B., and Brooks, G.R. (1993). Organizations Reacting to Hyperturbulence. In G. P. Huber and W. H. Glick (Ed.), *Organizational change and redesign: ideas and insights for improving performance* (pp. 66-111). New York: Oxford University Press.

Potter, R.H. (2003, October). Discharge Planning and Community Case Management for HIV-Infected Inmates: Collaboration Enhances Public Health and Safety. *Corrections Today*. pp. 80-82.

Roman, J., Townsend, W., and Bhati, A.S. (2003, July). Recidivism Rates for Drug Court Graduates: Nationally Based Estimates. The Urban Institute.

Samet, J.H., Mulvey, K.P., Zaremba, N., and Plough, A. (1999, May). HIV testing in substance abusers. *American Journal of Drug and Alcohol Abuse*. Retrieved April 8, 2004 from *http://www.findarticles.com/cf_dls/m0978/2_25/54724682/print.jhtml*

SAMHSA. (1997). National Household Survey on Drug Abuse: Population Estimates, 1996, p. 19, Table 2D).

SAMHSA. (2002, April 19). *Substance Abuse and Mental Health Services Administration, HIV/AIDS: Overview*. Retrieved April 20, 2004 from *http://search.samhsa. gov/...query=HIV+AIDS*

SAMHSA. (2004). *SAMHSA FY 2004 Budget: Government Performance Results Act Plan and Report (GPRA), 2.29 TCE: Community-based substance abuse treatment and HIV/AIDS outreach program*. Retrieved May 2, 2004 from *http://www.samhsa. gov/budget/content/2004/gpra/gpra2004-33.htm*

VIP Community Services. (1997, July 1). *Strategic Plan Revisited, Goals and Objectives*. Report of meeting.

Wilson, D.J. (2000, May). Drug Use, Testing, and Treatment in Jails. *Bureau of Justice Statistics Special Report*. Revised 9/29/00.

Culture, Community Networks, and HIV/AIDS Outreach Opportunities in a South Indian Siddha Organization

Kaylan Baban
Scott Ikeda
Deeangelee Pooran
Nils Hennig, MD, PhD
Debbie Indyk, PhD
Henry Sacks, MD, PhD
George Carter

SUMMARY. Background: Gandeepam is an NGO in rural south India, with an HIV prevalence rate estimated at 2-7 times the national average. Aside from several outreach programs, Gandeepam practices Siddha medicine. Objective: Evaluate Gandeepam's strengths and opportunities to promote HIV education. Design: Three weeks of observing clinic practice,

Kaylan Baban, Scott Ikeda, and Deeangelee Pooran, are Medical Students, and Nils Hennig, MD, PhD, Debbie Indyk, PhD, and Henry Sacks, MD, PhD are affiliated with the Mount Sinai School of Medicine, New York, NY. George Carter is affiliated with the Foundation for Integrative AIDS Research, New York, NY. Kaylan Baban is pursuing an MD/MPH at Mount Sinai School of Medicine.

Address correspondence to: Kaylan Baban, c/o Dr. Henry Sacks, One Gustave L. Levy Place, Box 1042, NY, NY 10029 (E-mail: Kaylan.Baban@mssm.edu).

[Haworth co-indexing entry note]: "Culture, Community Networks, and HIV/AIDS Outreach Opportunities in a South Indian Siddha Organization." Baban, Kaylan et al. Co-published simultaneously in *Social Work in Health Care* (The Haworth Press, Inc.) Vol. 42, No. 3/4, 2006, pp. 77-92; and: *The Geometry of Care: Linking Resources, Research, and Community to Reduce Degrees of Separation Between HIV Treatment and Prevention* (ed: Debbie Indyk) The Haworth Press, Inc., 2006, pp. 77-92. Single or multiple copies of this article are available for a fee from The Haworth Document Delivery Service [1-800-HAWORTH, 9:00 a.m. - 5:00 p.m. (EST). E-mail address: docdelivery@haworthpress.com].

meeting patients, and discussing organizational structure. A survey of attitudes toward HIV was completed. Results: Gandeepam reaches a broad cross-section of its community, and effectively disseminates information. No primary HIV prevention efforts were observed. Conclusion: Current strengths include an established network for information dissemination, and a strong community reputation. Tremendous social obstacles for disseminating effective HIV prevention messages remain. *[Article copies available for a fee from The Haworth Document Delivery Service: 1-800-HAWORTH. E-mail address: <docdelivery@haworthpress.com> Website: <http://www.HaworthPress.com> © 2006 by The Haworth Press, Inc. All rights reserved.]*

KEYWORDS. HIV, AIDS, prevention, education, community, India, Siddha

Siddha medicine is a healing method indigenous to south India, rooted in the Hindu religion, and based upon herbal, mineral, metal, and animal product treatments (Bin Mohammed, Abdul Raheem, & Kaivalyam, 1985; Ramamuthi, 1933; Weiss, 2003). This investigation was conducted as part of a preliminary assessment of Gandeepam, a traditional Siddha HIV/AIDS treatment facility in a poor rural region of the south Indian state of Tamil Nadu. This assessment was designed to guide the planning stages of a collaborative effort between Gandeepam and Mount Sinai School of Medicine in New York City, to conduct a controlled clinical trial of Gandeepam's herbal HIV/AIDS treatment. This project is an international twist on the new geometry of care (Rier & Indyk, this volume), defining the "vanguard" of HIV treatment as the community-based practice of traditional medicine, which can both inform and be informed by a more Western approach. Within this context, this paper presents a case-study that explores the ways in which linkages between a local, embedded community outreach organization, a traditional medical center, and a Non-Governmental Organization (NGO) with over 60 member community-based organizations, can pioneer a new approach to HIV treatment and prevention in rural communities in India. The paper begins by explaining the context within which Gandeepam operates, and its approaches to HIV treatment and prevention. Then the paper outlines Gandeepam's current successes (in collaboration with its partner NGOs) in integrating services and mobilizing community members–in domains other than HIV services. Finally, the paper explains why identifying traditional-practice collaboration partners such as Gandeepam is critical to the creation of HIV prevention and treatment programs in international contexts, and describes how the Gandeepam model might be extended to include HIV prevention.

WHAT IS GANDEEPAM?

Gandeepam is a non-governmental organization (NGO) practicing the south Indian tradition of Siddha medicine in the state of Tamil Nadu, and dedicated to improving the overall well-being of the rural community surrounding its base in Kilavayal village. The organization is named after the weapon known in Hindu lore as a gandeepam, sent by the god Shiva to the hero Arjuna to fight the evils of the world. However, despite the unilateral approach of its namesake, this organization does not rely upon just one weapon, but uses many approaches to empower its neighbors and root out the injustices rampant in rural India. Gandeepam offers not only affordable Siddha medical care for all who seek it, but also low-cost herbal gardens for home use, after-school tutorial programs for children, programs to help end child labor and women's self help groups.

In addition to these local efforts and accomplishments, Gandeepam is also the founding member of the Gandeepam Global Foundation (GGF), an association of 60 NGOs that among them cover almost all regions of Tamil Nadu state. Although the two organizations (Gandeepam and the GGF) are different entities by virtue of the GGF's inclusion of 59 other NGOs–many of which hold beliefs and values that differ widely from Gandeepam's and each other's–all 60 share goals of alleviating suffering and poverty in their regions, Gandeepam is the primary force steering the GGF, and there exists a great deal of overlap in the work and leadership of the two organizations. Therefore the work of the GGF member organizations is closely related to that of Gandeepam itself, and will be described below.

HEALTHCARE IN SOUTH INDIA

As in the rest of the country, healthcare in south India is dichotomized into "traditional" and "Western" systems, with a long history of tension that still often exists between the two (Hausman, 2002). Though the state and national governments now favor the allopathic model, the "Western" system of understanding and treating disease was not officially recognized in Tamil Nadu state until the early 1970s (Hausman, 2002). Thus, like many other traditional Tamil healthcare providers, Gandeepam is a strictly Siddha organization, with no current treatment linkages to allopathic or government organizations, and little interest in forming them in the future. Particularly among poor rural populations, it is not uncommon for clinics such as Gandeepam's to be the only means of healthcare accessible to patients–either geographically or financially. In addition, though many in this population would prefer allopathic treatment were it possible (Sobhan, Kumar, Kumar, Ravi Kanth, Adarsha, Mohammad, & Washington, 2004), there is also a significant proportion that places greater trust in Siddha. These circumstances make collaboration with organizations like Gandeepam essential to the effectiveness of HIV primary and secondary prevention efforts.

THE INDIAN GOVERNMENT'S HIV TREATMENT AND PREVENTION MESSAGES

The Indian government is fairly vocal in warning of the perils of HIV infection, promoting condoms (though a television ban on such promotions was only recently lifted through a change in government) (Sharma, 2004), and encouraging allopathic treatment. Unfortunately, the actions that coincide with these messages are often poorly planned and lack a structure that would enhance their success (Mudur, 2004). For example, the government stated that all HIV-infected persons presenting themselves at a government hospital would receive free allopathic treatment for their disease. However, the National AIDS Control Organisation, which manages India's national HIV/AIDS control program, has handled its job very ineffectively. Only 46% of its approved allocation of 11.6 billion IR ($250 million) was spent in the first 4 years of the 5 year program (Mudur, 2004). One result is that little provision was made to supply government hospitals with appropriate medications or reimburse their expenses. In addition, the fact that many physicians share common prejudices and refuse to treat HIV-infected patients (a position that describes approximately 22% of doctors in Tamil Nadu) seems also to have been ignored (Mudur, 2004). By self-report of Gandeepam patients, and corroborated independently both by Gandeepam clinic staff, and by staff at the GGF member organization HEAL (Human Education and Action for Liberation) (personal communication, July 13, 2004), the result is that many of those who sought help at the government hospitals, often at great expense for travel and lost wages, were turned away, and once again left to their own devices.

The Indian government's program to provide condoms for distribution through local community organizations seems promising, but it appears to lack guidelines or regulations that would allow the tracking of how the condoms are distributed and to whom. The recent reversal of the television ban on condom promotion coincides with the shifting emphasis away from *free* distribution of condoms (as was policy during the ban, presumably due to limitations on advertising) to use of marketing channels that distribute condoms for a fee (Sharma, 2004). Evidence citing expense and embarrassment as top deterrents to condom use among urban south Indian men (Thomas, Rehman, Malaisamy, Dilip, Suhadey, Priyadarsini, Purushotham, & Swaminathan, 2004) indicates that cutting free distribution programs, even if they were poorly organized, is likely to result in decreased condom use, particularly in remote and impoverished rural regions. Such a possibility seems only to add to the importance of an accessible and effective HIV education and prevention campaign.

METHOD

Three weeks were spent with Gandeepam and its partner organizations, with a view toward defining approaches to HIV/AIDS prevention, specifically with regard to education messages, and integration of prevention into existing community programs. Our purpose was to identify strengths of the Gandeepam model and ways in which it might link with international HIV providers to promote HIV awareness, prevention, and treatment in their communities. Methods of data collection included observing clinic practice, meeting patients, and discussing organizational structure and clinic protocol with Gandeepam's clinicians and administrators. In addition, a survey of HIV/AIDS treatment and prevention attitudes was completed by 39 GGF partners. Chart review (Ikeda et al., 2005) and laboratory assessment were also conducted (Pooran et al., 2005).

RESULTS

The Gandeepam Model

Ironically, what makes Gandeepam a critical partner in defining a new geometry of care for HIV treatment and prevention is actually the work it does *outside* its activities as a medical provider. Gandeepam is a strong and well-recognized presence in the community. In addition to providing medical care to patients seen at the clinic in Kilavayal and at Gandeepam's satellite clinics,[i] a large portion of Gandeepam's time and staff are dedicated to education and empowerment programs. Gandeepam's non-medical efforts have five primary foci, organized into Community-Based Organizations (CBOs). Although Gandeepam itself maintains all five of these programs in its region, the other members of the GGF also run some or all of these programs in their own locations.

First, the Child Labor Project is currently comprised of 15 villages and approximately 1575 children ages 6 to 17. Child labor is a major unifying concern through the region. The Project aims to increase educational opportunities for children who are valuable assets in this farming community.

Second, the Farmers' Group targets men, a group which is often neglected in community-development activities. The focus is Gandeepam-led plant cultivation trainings. Third, the Kitchen Herbal Garden project is the most wide-spread of Gandeepam's five CBOs. Gandeepam itself oversees Kitchen Herbal Gardens in five districts, amounting to approximately 654 villages or 60,000 households. The Kitchen Herbal Garden is one program common to all GGF member NGOs. Contact is made through selected community members who receive 3 days of training at Gandeepam on the cultivation and medicinal use of herbal plants. They then return home to cultivate model gardens and promote their use in the villages.

Fourth, Sanjeevini is a women's group which was originally established as a Gandeepam project. This women's group is now an autonomous NGO, but it is still headquartered in the same building. Each chapter has a maximum membership of 20 women all below the poverty line, like an estimated one-third of Tamil Nadu's rural population (Mehta & Shah, 2002) and with no more than five chapters per village. Members' attention is focused on issues such as keeping teachers in regular attendance at local schools, drawing regional government attention to problems with the village water supply, and educating other parents against the practice of child labor. And finally, the Youth Club is a CBO theoretically open to both genders, it is predominantly composed of young men who have aged out of the Child Labor Project. This imbalance is at least partly due to the fact that young women of the same age are often already married and engaged with other responsibilities. Members of the Youth Club help keep up cleanliness in the schools, volunteer with the Child Labor Project and, where possible, establish and maintain libraries in village community halls.

Villages neighboring Kilavayal establish local chapters of these groups, with initial help from Gandeepam. Some villages have founded chapters of all five groups, while some have only founded a chapter of one of them, according to the needs and interest level of the villagers. Though each of these programs has specific goals and target populations, the unifying focus is encouraging group members to maintain communal savings–and thus avoid the potentially ruinous step of taking high-interest outside loans in the future (Menon, 2004). Taken together, these community-based organizations provide a forum for virtually every member of the village; by working in a complementary fashion, they can form a net to strengthen the self-reliance of a village as a whole.

Structure and Influence of the Organization

At the time of the assessment, over 60,000 individuals were members of various components of this organization. The NGO hopes to expand its net to include a significant part of Tamil Nadu through this approach. Gandeepam offers a unifying theme–education and financial stability, but it is crucial to assess not only the breadth of participation, but also the extent of Gandeepam's influence over these groups.

When expanding to a new village, each program uses a similar template to recruit and organize its members: Gandeepam representatives approach the elected village president (or another prominent village member known to Gandeepam) and request permission to introduce their organization at a village meeting. These meetings are a normal part of village life, and are often held in the evenings, after work, so that as many villagers as possible can attend. Gandeepam representatives gauge the level of interest among those present and proceed accordingly. Therefore, using a method supported by many in India as the most effective to gain trust and disseminate information (Mapara, 2004; Chatterjee, 2004), Gandeepam uses familiar faces and works within the established ways of the community to maximize its chance of a large and favorable response to its programs.

Should a village show interest in starting a chapter of one or all of these programs, it will operate under two levels of leadership, local and regional. Locally, the chapter will elect three officials: a president, vice-president, and treasurer. These officials oversee the group's meetings (which take place once or twice a month), activities, funds, and supplies. In addition, Village Development Councils are established at the level of the *panchayet*[ii] and consist of an elected representative from local chapters of each program, as well as the leader of the *panchayet*, a Gandeepam staff person, and other prominent community leaders. Importantly, trainings are offered by Gandeepam every three months, focusing on leadership skills, book-keeping, fundraising, and individuals' rights.[iii] Village Development Council members carry this information back to their chapters. Thus, this system provides an infrastructure that builds Gandeepam's credibility and trustworthiness in the community, and lends itself well to other educational opportunities, such as dissemination of HIV prevention messages in the future.

On a larger scale, a handful of Gandeepam Global Foundation (GGF) organizations serve as regional heads for their sections of Tamil Nadu, and help to organize other GGF members. GGF regional heads are in touch throughout the year, and representatives from all Gandeepam Global Foundation partners meet quarterly. Gandeepam itself serves as one of these regional heads, with a hierarchy that descends from the Director of Gandeepam, through the Program Coordinator specific to that CBO, to the District Coordinators, and finally, in the case of the Kitchen Herbal Gardens, to the local field staff and Village Resource Persons. Overall, this communication network serves to ensure that local program chapters do not become too isolated, from one another or from Gandeepam, and allows smooth dissemination of new information and trainings from one level to the next.

For the purposes of evaluating Gandeepam's direct community influence, it is important to note that a chapter's participation in the Gandeepam-organized leadership systems persists only as long as it takes for the chapter to be "completed." Estimates of how long this takes range from six months to four years and may depend on the CBO, but "completion" indicates that the chapter leaders and the Program Coordinator agree the chapter is sufficiently well established to be essentially self-sufficient. From that point forward, the chapter operates on its own and is only periodically visited by Gandeepam representatives, thus significantly narrowing the opportunity for outside influence and new training.

Achieving Results: The Gandeepam Community Networks in Action

Gandeepam's big picture objectives in the community focus on the education, empowerment, and well-being of village members. From young children's tutorial programs and efforts to reduce under-age labor, to Youth Clubs that seek to foster the next generation of village leaders, to Kitchen Herbal Gardens and farming groups that seek to boost the village economically, nutritionally, and medicinally, Gandeepam has sought to create a net that will protect and lift up every member of the community.

The one concrete theme currently over-arching the trainings provided to each CBO and embodying Gandeepam's big picture objectives is the focus on encouraging group members to maintain communal savings as a means to realize these goals. Village District Council trainings impart basic knowledge, such as how to open a bank account and maintain balanced records, which is then passed on to group members in the villages. A pre-requisite of membership in all of these groups is that each member sets aside some quantity of money each month, to be deposited in the chapter's group bank account. Group members may then loan money among themselves when needed, at an interest rate agreed upon by members.

The importance of this system is that, to some extent, it obviates the necessity of seeking potentially ruinous high-interest outside loans. In this drought-devastated region, the rising rate of suicide among desperately in-debt farmers is regularly reported in the news (Prabhu, 2003; Sainath, 2004; "Farmer's suicide," 2004). The apparent success of this Gandeepam-enforced modicum of financial stability, and decreased vulnerability to outside high-interest loans, has the ability to fundamentally change the way that community members view their circumstances. They are now better equipped to help themselves and others, and not to view as inevitable the potentially ruinous debts that often drive struggling farmers to such drastic extremes.

Through this focus, Gandeepam seems to have identified a fundamental problem affecting all community members, and has used its leadership hierarchy to educate, and to enable community members to envision a solution and the means to achieve it. This is a model with the potential to do tremendous good if applied to the task of HIV education.

The Untackled Issue: Gandeepam and Combating the Spread of HIV

In light of the inspiring efficacy of Gandeepam's community model in mobilizing villagers and combating the attendant evils of poverty, it is singularly unfortunate that HIV/AIDS education is conducted almost entirely separately from Gandeepam's established community groups. Despite Gandeepam's avowed goal to eliminate HIV from Tamil Nadu state within ten years (a goal shared with the GGF), the responsibility for attaining that goal appears to fall solely to Gandeepam's clinic personnel, who operate within an entirely different and far less extensive model of community interaction than that previously described.

There is a great deal of stigma, fear, and even hatred surrounding an Indian villager infected with HIV (Sobhan et al., 2004). Gandeepam patients whose status is known to their neighbors have reported being pelted with stones when attempting to use the village water pump, receiving a barrage of verbal abuse, and being unable to find willing husbands for their daughters. Though the Indian government has engaged in what amounts to a media blitz, painting commercial trucks with the advice to "Avoid AIDS," and nailing signs to trees encouraging condom use, the subject remains largely taboo among the general public. Fear of the disease, and the almost equal fear of any intimation that they themselves may be infected, combines with a deep-rooted cultural unwillingness to discuss matters of sexual health, a topic that is very difficult to broach.

It therefore may not be a surprise that, far from the proactive approach taken to establishing CBO chapters in local villages, Gandeepam's clinic focuses on Siddha herbal treatment of existing disease, not prevention, and largely relies upon Gandeepam's word-of-mouth reputation to lead prospective patients to their Siddha practitioners. There are occasional circumstances in which a community member mentions an ill person to clinic field staff, who then make visits to that person's home in an effort to encourage them to seek Gandeepam's medical help. The fruitfulness of such methods of patient recruitment is unclear but, in a region where HIV infection carries as heavy a stigma as it does in rural Tamil Nadu, the risks involved in drawing attention to such an individual without their consent are likely to at least be on par with the potential benefits, and must be seriously considered.

Testifying further to Gandeepam's potential as an important HIV education and prevention organization, Gandeepam field staff have been known to conduct educational interventions upon request, when HIV-infected patients experience harassment from neighbors. These interventions consist of a visit to the patient's village, and discussion with their neighbors about the modes of transmission of HIV—often stressing, for example, that the virus cannot be contracted by sharing a water pump or other such interactions (according to one study, only 20% of India's general population knows that "HIV could not be transmitted through mosquito bites and shared meals") (Mudur, 2004). Effectiveness of these interventions in educating villagers about HIV and its transmission is unclear, but anecdotal evidence suggests that harassment does subside.

Gandeepam's HIV Treatment and Prevention Messages

Due to the lack of success of the Indian government's HIV treatment initiative and the prohibitive expense of allopathic treatments offered through other sources (Sainath, 2004), many HIV-infected Indians who prefer allopathic treatment (estimated by one study to be approximately 48% of Tamil Nadu's rural population) (Sobhan et al., 2004) join their more traditional neighbors and seek help from treatment models such as Siddha. A number of Gandeepam's HIV patients reported having begun allopathic treatment which they were forced to quit due to expense, or in fact never starting such a regimen in the first place due to lack of funds. An incomplete understanding of options seems also to have affected treatment decisions, as in the case of a majority of Gandeepam's Namakkal patients who were apparently unaware of a local NGO reportedly offering free allopathic HIV treatment.

These factors, combined with a preference for Siddha treatment that exists among a portion of the community (Hausman, 2002) mean that Gandeepam serves as a primary source of information and treatment for many Tamilians. As such, it is important to understand Gandeepam's beliefs and practices regarding HIV prevention and treatment. In contrast to the Indian government, Gandeepam's official message discourages the use of both condoms and allopathic medicines. Anti-retroviral therapy and other allopathic treatments are regarded as ineffective and unnecessarily harmful in their side-effects. Given such beliefs, it is not surprising that Gandeepam instead promotes its own treatment, an herbal blend believed to cure the patient, not just treat them, and to do so without side-effects. Gandeepam also discourages its HIV patients from engaging in sexual intercourse during treatment–the reason is not to prevent transmission, however, but rather a belief that intercourse hinders the patient's ability to fight the infection.

In summary: Gandeepam discusses HIV only with those who present themselves to the clinic already infected, patients are instructed to abstain from sex during treatment, and are considered cured once treatment is complete. The unfortunate result is that Gandeepam, a primary health and education resource for a large portion of Tamil Nadu, has not identified a need to educate against contraction or transmission of the virus.

Gandeepam Global Foundation's HIV Treatment and Prevention Messages

In contrast with Gandeepam itself, the 59 other organizations which, with Gandeepam, comprise the Gandeepam Global Foundation represent different regions of Tamil Nadu, and have varied and sometimes conflicting goals and belief systems. Some of the GGF member organizations have primarily Christian missions, some Hindu-influenced Siddha missions (like Gandeepam), and some are secular and admit to recommending Siddha treatment only as a last resort. However, they all share those goals identified earlier as Gandeepam's big-picture objectives in the community: raising the education, empowerment, and well-being of community members. The concrete form this agreement takes is the Kitchen Herbal Garden project; by addressing nutritional, economic, and medicinal needs, it has something for all parties regardless of strength of belief in Siddha practice. Therefore, the Kitchen Herbal Garden is the one project common to all 60 GGF NGOs.

A related but untapped unifying goal is the eradication of HIV from Tamil Nadu. Reflecting their different values and beliefs, however, discussions with GGF member organizations, as well as results of a survey of those members' attitudes towards HIV/AIDS,[iv] yielded widely varied approaches to education and prevention. Across the board, there was no discernible coordination with treatment.

Like Gandeepam, most GGF NGOs neither provide, promote, nor believe in condoms to prevent HIV transmission. Indeed, most are reluctant to discuss sexual health issues with men (who are not believed open to such dialogue) or single women (to whom cultural norms dictate that such dialogue is not relevant). Thus, those organizations that do promote condoms usually target married women. This intervention is unlikely to effect concrete change in the rising rate of HIV infection (Sobhan et al., 2004). A small number of GGF organizations do provide condoms to sex workers. The GGF partner organizations that participate in condom distribution do so using free latex condoms supplied by the national government; it is unclear how the proposed phasing-out of that system will affect these programs. Though promising, the details of these programs need further investigation.

CONCLUSIONS AND LOOKING FORWARD

Based on time spent with Gandeepam staff, patients, and partner organizations, it appears that Gandeepam has created a very large and influential education and empowerment network in its region, both locally on its own, and on a state level through its partners in the GGF. However–although fighting the spread of HIV is one of Gandeepam's and the GGF's top priorities–neither HIV education, nor treatment, nor prevention is among the goals of any of Gandeepam's five very successful CBOs. Issues concerning HIV/AIDS are dealt with separately by Gandeepam's clinic staff through treatment of infected patients, and do not involve discussions of how to prevent HIV transmission.

Thus, though in a unique position to raise awareness and combat the spread of HIV, it appears that Gandeepam, as well as its partners, are missing opportunities to do so, in part due to lack of integration of HIV education into its other programs that have already proven effective. As indicated in conversation with Gandeepam staff and survey responses from GGF members, this approach seems at least partly informed by local belief systems and cultural values that stigmatize both HIV/AIDS and frank discussions of sexual health.

In recognition of the different beliefs held by the parties at Gandeepam and Mount Sinai School of Medicine, the following realistically attainable goals are proposed: (a) Identify missed opportunities for integrating HIV prevention and treatment messages into Gandeepam's strategic and multiple programs to reduce local stigma against HIV patients, (b) Find ways to create a dialogue with Gandeepam about the concept of HIV prevention. To date, they have focused on treating those who present with a diagnosis. The NGOs are strategically positioned to talk about these issues, but there is a wide spectrum of beliefs and norms which currently continue to dichotomize HIV prevention and treatment.

This can be done by building upon Gandeepam's strength. In much the same way that book-keeping practices are passed down from Gandeepam through the members of the Village District Council to benefit individual villagers and help ward off debt, so too could such an educational program be initiated regarding HIV. Working within the established and proven system, the quarterly trainings at Gandeepam could begin to include HIV education messages to be carried home to local chapters. Such an effort would have the potential to reduce the stigma associated with HIV and perhaps even begin to curb the rising rate of infection.

The Gandeepam model is proven in the case of building financial stability, and shows great promise for HIV education and prevention. Like exorbitant debt among farmers, HIV is a life-threatening problem of growing magnitude, with the potential to impact all residents of Gandeepam's catchment area. Studies have shown that, particularly in the age group under 30, most Indians receive their information regarding HIV/AIDS from their peers, whom they trust (Sobhan et al., 2004; Thomas et al., 2004). A model such as that described for Sanjeevini or the Kitchen Herbal Gardens, wherein information begins at Gandeepam and moves incrementally closer to the members of an individual village chapter, lends itself perfectly to taking advantage of this circumstance; the basis of that system is that everyone involved has a personal relationship with those above and below them in the chain. Proactive education in the villages, conducted as a matter of course and independent of specific individuals, could make life much easier for HIV positive villagers, and better educate villagers to protect themselves and others from the spread of HIV.

On the subject of condoms: Given our strongly held belief–based on laboratory and epidemiological evidence (Carey, Herman, Retta, Rinaldi, Herman, & Athey 1992; Centers for Disease Control [CDC], 1988)– that latex condoms do reduce the transmission of HIV, Gandeepam's active discouragement of their use is a matter of great importance. Evidence, such as new pregnancies and remarriage in the course of treatment, indicates that not all Gandeepam patients are abstinent during treatment. Given that a chart review conducted concurrently with this investigation demonstrates that 68.8% of patients were shown by ELISA to be HIV positive on presentation (Ikeda et al., 2005), a significant risk that patients are transmitting the virus while in treatment can be concluded (post-treatment HIV viral load measurements are not available to demonstrate or refute continued risk). This can perhaps serve as a talking point on the subject between Gandeepam and Mount Sinai. Due in part to moral and religious concerns, it is not expected that Gandeepam will begin to promote condoms, but in the face of such evidence of continued sexual intercourse during treatment, perhaps Gandeepam may not continue to actively discourage their use.

Similar concerns on the part of the Mount Sinai investigators also apply to the question of Gandeepam's propagation of a negative attitude towards allopathic treatment of HIV/AIDS. Any number of approaches to increasing and encouraging rural Indian access to anti-retroviral drugs and other treatments is worthy of serious discussion. However, because of strong resistance to treatment linkages with allopathic or government organizations, in addition to the basic logistics of limited staffing capacity and inadequate access to laboratories that meet an international standard (Pooran et al., 2005), it unfortunately appears extremely improbable that Gandeepam is the appropriate vehicle for such plans. As the strongest known presence in its community, Gandeepam has unparalleled access to a region in desperate need of HIV education. This need is not yet being filled, but the potential is there. All evidence suggests that Gandeepam has a strong structure and outstanding potential to positively impact HIV/AIDS education and prevention in its community. If Gandeepam and Mount Sinai School of Medicine continue their working relationship, the proposed goals can serve as compromises through which to reduce the degrees of separation that currently exist within and among the collaborating communities. If instituted, building on Gandeepam's local and regional infrastructure, these practices could significantly benefit the state of HIV education and prevention in Tamil Nadu.

NOTES

i. For the purposes of this paper, the clinic in Namakkal, with its high volume of HIV patients, is most notable.

ii. A municipality that encompasses 10-15 villages.

iii. This last portion incorporates lawyers invited from outside Gandeepam.

iv. Survey written and administered to representatives of 39 GGF NGOs during a quarterly conference in July 2004.

REFERENCES

Bin Mohammed, A., Abdul Raheem, K. P., & Kaivalyam, K. (1985). The role of traditional healers in the provision of health care and family planning services: Ayurveda and sidda. *Malaysian Journal of Reproductive Health, 3*(1 Suppl.), S95-9.

Carey, R. F., Herman, W. A., Retta, R. S., Rinaldi, J.E., Herman, B. A., & Athey, T. W. (1992). Effectiveness of latex condoms as a barrier to human immunodeficiency virus-sized particles under conditions of simulated use. *Sexually Transmitted Diseases, 19*(4), 230-40.

Centers for Disease Control and Prevention. (1988). Condoms for prevention of sexually transmitted diseases. *MMWR Morbidity and Mortality Weekly Report, 37*, 133-137.

Chatterjee. (2004). HIV/AIDS prevention carries on in rural India. *The Lancet: Infectious Diseases, 4*, 386.

Farmer's suicide rocks the house again. (2004, July 15). *The Hindu.*

Hausman, G. J. (2002). Making medicine indigenous: Homeopathy in south india. *Social History of Medicine, 15*(2), 303-322.

Ikeda, S., Baban, K., Pooran, D., Hennig, N., Carter, G., Indyk, D., & Sacks, H. (2005). *Assessment and Review of HIV Positive Patient Medical Records from a Traditional Siddha Medicine Hospital in Tamil Nadu, India.* Unpublished manuscript.

Mapara, E. M. (2004). No 'lack of human resources' and all are 'risk groups' [Letter to the editor]. *British Medical Journal, 329,* 252-b.

Mehta, A., & Shah, A. (2002). *Chronic poverty in India: overview study.* Retrieved January 13, 2005 from Chronic Poverty Research Centre, http://www.eldis.org/static/DOC106.htm

Menon, P. (2004, November 19).An agrarian crisis. *The Hindu.*

Mudur, G. (2004). Audit report criticizes India's slow progress on AIDS. *British Medical Journal, 329*:252.

Pooran, D., Hennig, N., Baban, K., Ikeda, S., Indyk, D., Carter, G., & Sacks, H. (2005). *Needs Assessment Study Establishing a Scientific Study of Siddha Medicine Treatments of HIV/AIDS.* Unpublished manuscript.

Prabhu, N. (2003, September 3).Failures on many fronts behind farmers' suicide. *The Hindu.*

Ramamuthi, I. (1933). *The hand book of Indian medicine or the gems of Siddha system.* Erode: Sri Vani Vilas Press.

Sainath, P. (2004, July 1). Anatomy of health disaster. *The Hindu.*

Sharma, D.C. (2004). India reverses policy on condom advertising. *The Lancet: Infectious Diseases, 4,* 538.

Sobhan, K., Kumar, T. S., Kumar, G. S., Ravi Kanth, R., Adarsha, A., Mohammad, A. S., & Washington, R. (2004). HIV and AIDS-Awareness and attitudes among males in a rural population. *Indian Journal of Community Medicine, 29*(3), 141-2.

Thomas, B.E., Rehman, F., Malaisamy, M., Dilip, M., Suhadey, M., Priyadarsini, P., Purushotham, N. K., & Swaminathan, S. (2004). A study of condom acceptability among men in an urban population in south India. *AIDS and Behavior, 8*(2), 215-20.

Weiss, R. S. (2003). The reformulation of a holy science: Siddha medicine and tradition in South India. (Doctoral dissertation, University of Chicago, 2003). *Dissertation Abstracts International, 64/07,* 2529.

Requisites, Benefits, and Challenges of Sustainable HIV/AIDS System-Building: Where Theory Meets Practice

Debbie Indyk, PhD
David A. Rier, PhD

SUMMARY. This paper is the third and final of a series that has previously presented the rationale (Rier and Indyk, this volume) and major program elements (Indyk and Rier, this volume) of an approach to link community and tertiary sociomedical providers, clients/patients, sites, and systems into an integrated response to HIV/AIDS. The primary goal has been to improve sociomedical HIV/AIDS services for a hard-to-reach inner city population. The current paper first summarizes the main advantages (e.g., greater efficiency; more realistic, effective programs with greater credibility among the community; stimulation of knowledge production and dissemination amongst players rarely formally engaged in such activities; creation of a platform useful for other applications) of this work. It then examines some of the main organizational challenges in conducting the work (involving issues such as personnel, coordination, funding, turf conflicts, sustainability). From this discussion emerge organ-

Debbie Indyk, PhD, is affiliated with the Mount Sinai School of Medicine, New York, NY. David A. Rier, PhD, is affiliated with Bar-Ilan University, Ramat-Gan, Israel.

[Haworth co-indexing entry note]: "Requisites, Benefits, and Challenges of Sustainable HIV/AIDS System-Building: Where Theory Meets Practice." Indyk, Debbie, and David A. Rier. Co-published simultaneously in *Social Work in Health Care* (The Haworth Press, Inc.) Vol. 42, No. 3/4, 2006, pp. 93-110; and: *The Geometry of Care: Linking Resources, Research, and Community to Reduce Degrees of Separation Between HIV Treatment and Prevention* (ed: Debbie Indyk) The Haworth Press, Inc., 2006, pp. 93-110. Single or multiple copies of this article are available for a fee from The Haworth Document Delivery Service [1-800-HAWORTH, 9:00 a.m. - 5:00 p.m. (EST). E-mail address: docdelivery@haworthpress.com].

izational requisites to conducting this work (e.g., development of key boundary-spanning figures; attention to the specific interests of potential linkage partners; translation efforts to demonstrate the value of participation; a continuous quality improvement approach featuring wide distribution of feedback in user-friendly form; flexibility, tact and patience), so that others can adapt and apply the linkage approach to manage HIV/AIDS or other problems. Finally, we explain how theory and practice have driven one another in this work. *[Article copies available for a fee from The Haworth Document Delivery Service: 1-800-HAWORTH. E-mail address: <docdelivery@haworthpress.com> Website: <http://www.HaworthPress.com> © 2006 by The Haworth Press, Inc. All rights reserved.]*

KEYWORDS. AIDS services, inter-organizational linkages, sustainability, knowledge production and dissemination

The papers in this section have presented a theoretical rationale for a new "geometry of care," (Rier & Indyk), and have provided a series of case examples illustrating the application of this approach to the development of integrated sociomedical HIV/AIDS services (outreach, prevention, treatment, and support), especially for high-risk, hard-to-reach populations. This approach is grounded in the premise that not only academic researchers and clinicians, but also community-based clinicians and service providers, and clients/patients as well, possess unique expertise that makes them vital participants in generating, disseminating, and applying knowledge for fighting the AIDS epidemic. The approach requires the construction, maintenance, and continuing renovation of the infrastructure needed to generate and sustain the changing inter-organizational linkages required among and between community, medical center, and patients/clients. These linkages, in turn, are built up to create webs, in which each party or site serves as a hub for consuming, producing, and transmitting its unique knowledge and insights throughout the system.

In this paper, we take a step back to assess the work. First, we consider the key benefits of this approach, and consider its contribution to the provision of comprehensive, integrated care. Second, we describe some of the organizational and other challenges encountered, and (third), distill from this discussion some of the organizational requisites for performing such work. We acknowledge that putting the new geometry of care into practice is complicated, arduous, and often thankless work. This paper is designed to anticipate and draw attention to some of the key challenges that this work presents and, in so doing, assist individuals and organizations in preparing to meet them.

BENEFITS

As discussed in a previous article (Rier & Indyk) in this volume, the new geometry of care yields several benefits. These are summarized in Figure 1. First, this approach helps the medical center to reach and serve high-risk, hard-to-reach populations. In parallel, it extends and expands the scope of community-based organizations' (CBOs) services. More generally, it brings coherence to the often chaotic delivery of services, and makes maximal use of scarce resources. It also means that interventions of all sorts are better suited to the needs and constraints of their target populations, and more credible in their eyes.

This last point, in particular, is due partly to a specific strength of this linkage approach—it puts into circulation the knowledge, insights, and experiences of community-based providers, and even of the clients and patients they serve (Rier & Indyk, this volume). Otherwise, such input would rarely reach beyond the local community. In fact, through the linkage approach, service providers such as community-based social workers or needle-exchange staff sometimes even engage in formal knowledge-dissemination activities such as preparing and presenting papers at conferences, and writing for scholarly journals. Recognizing frontline providers as researchers, harvesting the fruits of their expertise, and applying them to service, treatment, and research, represent key benefits of the approach, and may ultimately prove its most lasting contribution.

In describing this approach, we emphasize knowledge production, evaluation, and dissemination, but more than this is involved. Beyond circulation of insights, this approach also helps extract maximal benefit from the social contacts and connections available at each party's particular social location. Uniting such diverse players for a common goal thus mobilizes a breadth of various forms of social capital far greater than what any one type of actor could marshal on his/her own (of course, it also raises turf issues and other conflicts, as discussed below).

There is another level to this work. Just as the new geometry of care unites community and medical center *providers* for improved service delivery, so it integrates the *functions* of prevention, education, service, and evaluation which, for too long in the AIDS epidemic, were viewed as wholly distinct. Our integrating approach, by contrast, can create ser-

FIGURE 1. Benefits of the Linkage Approach

INFRASTRUCTURE

♦ *Link actors and functions*

•Actors:
   •Frontline community providers
   •Academic clinicians
   •Researchers
   •Community and medical center administrators
   •Patients/Clients

•Functions:
   •Prevention
   •Treatment
   •Service
   •Education
   •Research

♦ *We hard-wired the system: It can carry any traffic, to address other issues, e.g.:*
   •Substance abuse
   •TB
   •Breast cancer

CONCRETE

♦ *Reached and engaged many inner-city residents into:*
   •Prevention
   •Service
   •Treatment
   •Education

♦ *Community input = more realistic, credible interventions*
♦ *Collaborative evaluation model*
♦ *Developed multiple funding streams*
♦ *Maximal return from scarce resources*

vices designed so that clients coming into a CBO for help with immigration problems can also receive information about AIDS prevention, or be referred to AIDS testing. Our work (Indyk & Rier, this volume) demonstrates that prevention, education, and behavior change must occupy a key role in interventions and programs at *each* point on the continuum of treatment and service–rather than being compartmentalized into discrete, isolated units. Linkage is especially critical to prevention, since this requires individuals to change their behaviors. Without close contact and input from at-risk individuals and their providers, prevention interventions have only limited success.

Finally, let us consider the wider implications of the infrastructure created through this approach. This infrastructure consists primarily of mechanisms such as various educational forums, technical assistance agreements, collaborations to perform research and cultivate funding streams, referral agreements, and network-building to link community providers with medical center providers, and with those each serves. The development of this web of linkages, collaboration, and knowledge transfer brings two advantages: one "micro" and one "macro."

On the micro level, this approach reaches more underserved, high-risk individuals and engages them in networks of HIV/AIDS treatment, services, and prevention. Moreover, the new geometry of care insures that, once thus engaged, the mechanisms and relationships *already exist* with which to work on *other* sociomedical problems, beyond those (such as substance abuse) directly related to HIV/AIDS. These might include employment, housing, mental health, hypertension, etc.

What is true for the individual client brought into a service relationship is equally true on the macro level. Through the linkages this work generates, the approach essentially "wires the system," creating a potential platform for addressing multiple sociomedical ills. Too often, however, the wiring is only bi-directional. Wiring is needed to link central and peripheral networks to unite community, public health providers, and medical care providers. Thus wired, this system can carry numerous types of traffic, since much of the same wiring can be utilized to address problems of engagement, assessment, treatment, and evaluation. For example, our experience collaborating with one CBO, Dominican Sisters Family Health Service (DSFHS) (Indyk & Rier, this volume), demonstrates that the same CBO that provides basic HIV/AIDS support services is also a strategic setting in which to reach individuals at different stages of awareness, engagement, and management of tuberculosis (TB), mental illness, diabetes, and heart disease. Many of the practitioners with whom DSFHS interacts belong to overlapping professional communities. However, they tend to compartmentalize and suppress their multiple identities, thus missing opportunities to forge common ground with their colleagues. Mental health practitioners, drug treatment practitioners, and HIV providers are often, independently, treating the same clients. Yet it has taken the input from grassroots providers (employing their own overlapping ties) via multiple top-down networks to bring these discrete systems together.

The expertise and infrastructure developed around inner-city AIDS are particularly adaptable to prevention problems, such as substance abuse and TB, for which risk reduction–*hence the community and pa-*

tient–are key. HIV and AIDS in the inner city are partly the product of the poverty and related conditions that are also at the root of problems such as substance abuse. Indeed, substance abuse is the primary cause of AIDS in the inner city, either directly, by sharing of infected needles when injecting heroin or cocaine, or indirectly, by sexual transmission from those infected through needle-sharing. Similarly, the pattern of the spread of TB in the inner city closely follows that of HIV, as it is also linked with poverty and its correlates. As linkage work evolved, there arose a strategic opportunity to integrate substance abuse and TB into AIDS network activities, since there was growing awareness of the significant overlap in both the individuals at risk, and the providers involved in responding to these problems. Regarding TB, for example, CBOs are particularly well positioned for direct observational therapy (DOT), the best way to manage TB for these patients. Medical center providers may know which drugs to use, but the CBO is best at *finding* patients, and ensuring they actually take their medication. Indeed, one result of the linkage approach has been a preventive form of DOT (DOPT) for high-risk individuals reached at needle exchange programs.

In one example of the integration of AIDS with substance abuse work, we have brought primary and secondary prevention (an approach which the Centers for Disease Control and Prevention [CDC] currently endorses strongly) closer together (Strauss, this volume). This unites a group of providers who are working with the same clients but at different geographic locations, focusing on different problems with different expertise (and often reaching individuals at different stages of risk and disease). From this work, we learned that the HIV+ individuals in need of (secondary prevention) treatment with anti-retroviral therapy *also* need primary prevention support to reduce risk of acquiring other infections and diseases.

Furthermore, our work with various modalities of drug treatment providers made it clear that, though primary and secondary addiction prevention have much in common, these were normally not linked to one another. Primary prevention requires engagement and motivation of the target to support the behavioral goal. Historically, primary prevention was offered through targeted educational campaigns employing outreach workers. Secondary prevention was offered through treatment sites where retention in treatment was often a measure of successful outcome. However, as various providers worked with the same populations at various points along the continuum of their exposure to drugs and disease, many frontline providers recognized that education, alone, did little to alter behavior. Clients needed to be reached and offered messages matching their stage of readiness to accept, execute, and sustain targeted behavior. Treatment providers also realized that, when individuals dropped out of treatment or relapsed, they needed to be re-engaged. In both instances, individuals need to be met where they are, and offered an array of primary and secondary prevention services suiting their vulnerability and disease profile.

The linkage approach is potentially valuable for any serious problem affecting marginalized communities in which prevention, early intervention, and sociomedical management are important. Such problems include hypertension, diabetes, cancer, heart disease, etc. Medical centers may be able to offer powerful treatments, interventions, or even cures, but they cannot provide them to those who fail to enter the system before their disease has advanced beyond effective reach of such measures. Alone, medical centers can do even less about preventing these problems' occurrence or progression, or even early detection and early intervention.

For example, breast cancer can often be managed effectively, if detected early. Public health campaigns may stimulate such early detection in middle class communities, but often fail to reach the most marginalized members of the inner city, for whom paying the rent is more immediate a concern than mammography. *But*, if the CBO that helps women secure rent subsidies *also* could help arrange (through medical center referral agreements) mammograms for them, early detection and effective treatment are possible. The CBOs are best suited to identify and provide the requisites for chemotherapy follow-up–the childcare and carfare which can make the difference between remaining in care and dropping out. Moreover, effective linkages to those in charge of the mammography program at the medical center could allow the CBOs to transmit the sort of details about their clients' problems and priorities which could lead to better, more realistic outreach programs. Careful case management can help walk clients through the various services they need, vastly improving ultimate outcomes. Yet coordination is not enough. Given the complexity of these problems, effective action is virtually impossible without sustained input from those actually affected, another strength of the linkage approach.

CHALLENGES AND REQUISITES

Numerous obstacles exist in performing this linkage work. This section describes some of the key challenges encountered. From this discussion will emerge some possible responses, and a summary of key requisites for applying this approach elsewhere.

First, knitting together dozens of linkages at every conceivable type of node in the sociomedical care system–on both personal and institutional levels–is complex, labor intensive, and costly work. Ultimately, the existence of linkages may naturally stimulate additional cross-linkages and collaboration. Yet the initial process of laying in this wiring involves countless meetings, discussions, presentations, sessions of providing technical support, and other linkage devices. This process requires at least one actor (and preferably many) with sufficiently broad connections and credibility to enlist a critical mass of players with whom to push the work through its start-up phase.

Indeed, personnel issues are central to this work. To take just one challenge: how can we institutionalize the dedication and good will manifested by a very small number of key players? Often, a new program commands initial enthusiasm and support from important administrators who "champion" the work, motivate staff, and mobilize resources (Kraft, Mezoff, Sogolow et al., 2000). However, such support often wanes as difficulties develop and other priorities emerge (Sogolow, Kay, Doll et al., 2000), or if essential personnel leave. One start in addressing such problems would be to fund formal boundary-spanning positions. As was the case in the development of perinatal medicine (Indyk, 1987), figures with local and cosmopolitan ties to research, practice, teaching, and policy are crucial here. Likely candidates for such roles must be identified and cultivated for as many hubs as possible within the system. However, heavy reliance on specific individuals can create vulnerability. Therefore, existing linkages must be formalized and institutionalized wherever possible, lest the webs prove to be a house of cards, collapsing with the departure of a few founding personnel.

The problem of staff turnover has been particularly important over the years with HIV/AIDS. First, a number of important players have, themselves, had HIV/AIDS. As was the case with AIDS grassroots organizations (Indyk & Rier, 1993), especially prior to the advent of today's effective antiretroviral therapy, their bouts of illness or their eventual deaths have caused periodic disruptions in staff continuity. More recently, other researchers have also noted a form of "AIDS fatigue" amongst potential project staff, as well as the normal turnover characterizing many low-paying CBO positions (e.g., Chillag, Bartholow, Cordeiro et al., 2002; Kegeles, Rebchook, Hays et al., 2000; Rotheram-Borus, Rebchook, Kelly et al., 2000).

One basic obstacle is getting providers to recognize that they are inter-dependent with vastly different sectors of the health care system. Some academic providers need to be convinced that they have something to learn from non-MD social workers or outreach workers. Conversely, some community-based social service providers must overcome their mistrust and resentment of large medical centers (particularly when these have a reputation for unresponsiveness to the community) before they can recognize the benefits of collaboration with academic providers who often occupy privileged social locations of race and class. Thus, before collaboration is possible, academics must often convince community providers that they are sufficiently sensitive to the community, and seek not just to exploit a research opportunity and then move on. Community providers, meanwhile, must often convince the academics that they possess sufficient skills and professionalism to justify collaboration.

A related issue is the culture clash which often results when those of very different backgrounds and professional roles collaborate. The different environments of goals, incentives, and values within which community providers and academic researchers operate have already been noted as a source of culture clash in joint activities (Rotheram-Borus, Rebchook, Kelly et al., 2000). In our own experience, this has been a frequent source of misunderstanding, placing a premium on good communication and the careful cultivation of trust between collaborators.

Another problem is that extensive boundary spanning activities, while essential, may undermine the formal division of labor and lines of authority which can be critical to the smooth operation of complex organizations. Tensions exist between various types of providers even within the same setting, as well as between those of different settings. Without careful coordination and diplomacy, linkage work can lead to turf conflicts, such as when social work and nursing services pursue overlapping activities.

Competing interests and interpretations are predictable whenever so many boundaries are traversed (Freidenberg, 1991). For example, bringing together providers who treat sexually-transmitted diseases (STDs) with those working in HIV counseling led to serious turf issues and other conflicts. Implementing the insight that treating STDs (an example of secondary prevention) serves simultaneously as primary prevention of HIV, implied substantial changes in funding patterns and treatment modalities. Given their differing interests, these two communities differed in their enthusiasm for participating in such work. For the many reasons listed above, key personnel require tact, patience, and the ability to listen.

Moreover, the many participating agencies, departments, and programs require periodic reminders of what they gain through their collaboration, lest the complaint rise up, "What's in it for me, lately?" As has long been recognized in the social movements literature, those who feel they would reap the benefits even without their own labor might be tempted to be "free riders" (Olson, [1965]1971; Oliver, 1984). As a corollary, we should not expect participation motivated by altruism alone. To paraphrase an axiom of diplomacy: Providers and agencies have interests, not friends. That being the case, new linkage possibilities should be scrutinized for potential mutual benefit. Promising opportunities can be "marketed" by "translating" (Kraft, Mezoff, Sogolow et al., 2000) the appeal of the work into terms relevant to the specific individual, site, or system being solicited as a linkage partner.

However a degree of altruism, at least amongst key figures, *is* sometimes a distinct advantage. This is particularly because the institutional reward system (both in the community and medical center) has yet to "catch up" to this work. Too often, the system fails sufficiently to value shared work that diminishes or obliterates individual accomplishment. In another sphere, financing of boundary spanning activities is complicated by the disparate salary scales in community and academic settings and, especially, by frequent disagreement over allocation and control of resources.

More generally, funding has presented special challenges throughout this work. Traditionally, AIDS treatment and prevention funding sources have not allowed grants to be used to support agency-specific infrastructure development; monies have been restricted to support service delivery. An exception to this is limited Federal money distributed by states to support a network of AIDS providers. An example of this is the East Harlem HIV Care Network, one of fifteen networks serving high HIV prevalence communities in New York State.

The overall project began with a $600,000 grant from the Aaron Diamond Foundation to the first author. Covering the years 1990-94, these funds helped launch the initial work around infrastructure-building and community-based resource, program and data development, and evaluation. However, this was virtually the only funding given in direct support of the overall linkage work. Lacking a stable source of additional "dedicated" money, the continued sustenance and extension of this work has been forced to rely on a series of discrete grants that usually committed us to deliver specific services (e.g., to design and provide HIV training to a given number of health professionals at a given site). However, such funding did not allow for the fact that our ability to provide the proper education rested on our ability to offer linkages to diverse forms of resources. For instance, we have received grants to help CBOs better serve their clients by expanding their outreach and referral services. Yet the referral networks to which we link these CBOs are fruits of all the previous, little-recognized work invested in cultivating diverse providers and sites, and constructing linkage devices to bring them into contact with one another. Having done this, we are able to link them with the CBOs, to everyone's benefit. But precisely that capacity, in many ways the core value we offer, has seldom received direct support.

The work has thus been funded largely piecemeal, forcing us to divert enormous amounts of time to cobbling together support from various "soft-money" funding streams. Those replicating this approach would do well to seek "hard money" for linkage coordination, should such sources exist. In the longer term, the success of the work presented herein may help lead to more recognition and support from funding sources for the necessary infrastructure development.

The funding difficulties just described are partly related to a corollary, management-level issue. Much of our collaboration with CBOs has involved our assisting them to augment their programs by obtaining new grants (Indyk and Rier, this volume). Frequently, we were included in such funding, if at all, only as evaluators of the work. Though such "side" funding did help underwrite survival, it did not, as discussed above, directly support the underlying infrastructure/linkage development at the heart of the work. To a degree, the time and energy devoted to helping other organizations increase their funding came at the cost of our neglecting to devote sufficient resources to securing the direct types of funding our own work required. To that extent, at least, the altruism mentioned above must be tempered with the realism necessary to maintain the overall enterprise.

A whole separate category of challenges arises from the fact that the AIDS epidemic is a moving target. Over time, we have observed and participated in several types of shifts in the focus of the problem, which shifts have required ongoing reassessments and responses. Conversely, this work has evolved with time. It is an equal challenge to ensure that the changes in the nature of the response to AIDS articulate sufficiently with changes in the AIDS epidemic itself.

Locally, for example, certain changes with time are evident from attendance patterns at linkage functions. Thus, we have seen more chemical dependency programs join AIDS networks, as their work has converged with that of HIV service providers. Since such programs have few existing links to other providers, special efforts have been made to create such links. While top-down HIV and substance abuse agencies and networks have only recently begun to encourage integration and linkage to their counterparts, we have long been encouraging and supporting collaboration between groups and their linkage from the bottom-up, through informal forums and training. Many clinical providers initially were willing to deal with substance abuse as a treatment challenge only because they recognized that shared needles posed a major transmission route. They gained a broader perspective by working with groups of substance abuse providers who had originally come together to advocate for HIV services for the critical mass of users who were infected. In their view, the treatment model needed to be changed in order to engage and reach substance users "where they were at." By bringing together this diverse group of treatment specialists, who came from methadone, residential, and day program treatment "camps," individuals were able to select elements of their respective modalities and test them out informally. The boundaries among different treatment modalities have blurred enormously, enabling eclectic incorporation of strengths of each approach.

Another change in attendance patterns is that the seniority and authority of those attending linkage functions has declined with time. For example, the core group at meetings of the East Harlem HIV Care Network (a consortium of over 100 providers providing HIV-related services, brought together monthly to share information and develop linkages) was once dominated by decision-makers such as administrators, directors, and executives. Today, attendees come increasingly from among the front-line and direct service providers. This participation yields crucial input from those closest to our target populations. It also suggests that the linkage work is being normalized and routinized, and is not the experimental project of a handful of elites. However, front-line providers lack the authority to implement new policy, such as agreements for technical assistance, service referral, etc. Also, providers new to AIDS work are often sent to these meetings as a form of orientation, and not as part of their actual work. For linkage mechanisms such as the East Harlem HIV Care Network or community case rounds, which are coalitions of service providers, the challenge is to think constantly about who is coming–and who must be attracted and retained–in order to accomplish certain tasks. Are the people sitting around the table the *right* people for the task at hand? Do they provide or are they linked to the needed resources? Ideally, linkage programs would enjoy balanced participation among executive, rank-and-file, and consumer communities. Yet it is difficult to recruit and engage new participants unless the members are hospitable to new voices and tolerate the power shifts that may ensue.

All this suggests that, while institutionalization is vital to ensure sustainability, *flexibility* is also critical, particularly since it is "not possible to develop an intervention package that will, in all respects, retain a long shelf life" (Kegeles, Rebchook, Hays et al., 2000:71). While some programs simply reach the end of their life cycle, flexibility promotes the continued relevance of the work. Our approach assumes that, at any given point, the current picture stems from a specific confluence of needs, opportunities, and resources. These, in turn, represent but one phase in a shifting, evolving process. One example is the fate of our weekly AIDS Seminar series (Indyk and Rier, this volume). As it ceased to play an important role in person-to-person networking, attendance dropped off. Rather than cancel the series, we began to have it web-cast and archived. Thus, apart from the on-site, real-time audience, additional providers could log on at their convenience, from their own sites. This preserved the overall vitality of the series (until its funding terminated in 2003). As this experience shows, adaptability means the difference between *renovating* and *razing* organizational structures and linkage mechanisms.

Flexibility is built into the design due partly to the focus on continuous quality improvement and assessment (below). Moreover, the diversity of the linked parties, and the richness of the connections between them, have vastly improved feedback. This, in turn, has helped us respond swiftly to changes in the constellation of needs, opportunities, and challenges we face.

Flexibility plays another key role in this work. One seasoned front-line clinician/researcher likened her work to wearing a wide variety of "Post-It®" stickers, and inviting clients to peel off and use those stickers (i.e., services) they felt ready for. A client who will gladly accept rent subsidy assistance or help in arranging clinic visits may still balk at confronting issues raised by HIV counseling.

As with clients, so with systems and providers. Like clients, both providers and their organizations can become set in their ways, adhering to a limited, static view of their role. Frequently, they also face real limits on resources such as time, money, manpower, and skills base. A cash-strapped CBO might be so consumed by chasing money to continue existing services (Sogolow, Kay, Doll et al., 2000) that they lack time to consider the long-term value of collaboration in cultivating new funding streams. Building linkages requires coordinators prepared to offer a variety of menu options, allowing providers and organizations to select those assistance or collaboration opportunities they are prepared to pursue. This dovetails with the overall need, discussed above, to translate interventions into terms suitable to the goals, capacities, and orientations of organizations, in order to enroll them as enthusiastic participants and retain their support.

As with clients, systems, and providers, so with the linkage approach itself. The overall approach can be adapted, in whole or in part, as needs and resources dictate. The first author has applied the "stages of change" concept (Prochaska & DiClemente, 1986) to understand client, provider, and system barriers to change, and to develop matched interventions to execute and maintain change (Indyk, Coury-Doniger, Grosz et al., 1997). This might apply to a client beginning to consider lowering HIV risk by using clean syringes, or a network of CBOs and social service agencies deciding whether to link programs and resources with each other and with a medical school. Change on any level is rarely embraced instantly, and the approach is highly sensitive to this. The stages of change model reminds us that linkage work is a long-term process that must often be conducted gradually, with participants of all sorts being allowed insofar as possible to proceed at their own pace. This can help prevent miscommunication, and situations in which one side feels the other is dragging its feet, while the latter feels the former is trying to "railroad" through radical, destabilizing changes.

To continue to reach the hardest-to-reach, those currently lost even to CBOs, we must move even deeper into the community. Just as new spurs are added to an existing rail line, we have been cultivating new linkages, beyond CBOs, to programs that do (or could) reach them (Indyk, London, Tackley et al., 1998; London, Indyk, Clark et al., 1998). Thus, we have collaborated with a needle-exchange program, many of whose clients are not currently engaged by CBOs. Perhaps we will eventually add linkages to other street-level programs, and to prisons, to serve their high-risk populations.

On the other hand, sometimes internal linkage ("in-reach") is called for. Recently, at Mount Sinai, most new HIV patients have entered medical care as in-patients, rather than through community clinics. These individuals are not currently being reached early enough; they enter care only when already very sick, and usually lack any real history of primary care. These patients can at least be reached in the hospital. A proper post-discharge plan, including linkages to community-based sociomedical services, can prevent their being returned to the service void from which they entered.

A critical component of all the web-building work described herein is continuous quality improvement (Indyk, Belville, and Indyk, 1995). The Mount Sinai-DSFHS collaboration, for example, has featured joint development and expansion of a powerful, customized relational data management system enabling the CBO to track their clients and to improve their reporting capability (Indyk and Indyk, 1995). Access to user-friendly health data can be immensely empowering for CBOs and those they serve (Brown and Mikkelsen, 1990; Kroll-Smith and Floyd, 1997; Edelstein, 1988; McKnight, [1978]1990). Over the years, this has proven a particularly valuable tool in identifying clients' shifting needs.

For those interested in applying the linkage approach, the preceding discussion (along with Rier and Indyk and the other articles in this volume) yields some key organizational requisites. These are summarized in Figure 2.

"GROUNDED SERVICE": THE INTEGRATION OF THEORY AND PRACTICE

The papers in this volume present a new approach to the provision of HIV services–a new geometry of care that integrates disparate providers, agencies, and functions. The first section of this volume has provided several examples of this approach in action at a system level. Most importantly, a system-level implementation of this approach illustrates the functional complementarities of scale between community-based providers and the tertiary medical center. At the root of the linkages created by this approach is a commitment to diffusion of knowledge, and an appreciation of the unique expertise that each provider at each location in the sociomedical system can provide.

While the theoretical insight into the locus-embedded nature of expertise led to an emphasis on linkage in service design, the linkage work (practice), itself, generated its own theoretical insights. When we watched a community-based social service provider ask a question at a medical center seminar which showed him to be on the frontier of AIDS knowledge, when we heard an academic researcher state that he turned to a grassroots newsletter for the latest information on experimental AIDS treatments, when it was continually demonstrated to us how much community-based providers knew about the lives of those in the inner city–and how little those in teaching hospitals often knew–we understood that AIDS was bringing broad changes. Our work with CBOs prepared us to examine the case of grassroots AIDS treatment advocacy

FIGURE 2. Requisites of the Linkage Approach

1. Boundary-spanning activities to link practice settings, disciplines, and research between (and within) medical center and community-based programs.
2. Forums for knowledge exchange among hospital- and community-based providers.
3. Ideally, a central (tactful, patient) figure or figures to promote, execute, and monitor linkages.
4. Development of supervisory staff positions that facilitate overlapping roles in research, education, and practice within and between medical center- and community-based programs.
5. Mechanisms facilitating input from clients and patients.
6. Encouragement of frontline providers, and their clients/patients, to recognize their potential role as creators and disseminators of knowledge.
7. A critical mass of community and medical center personnel involved in planning.
8. Development of shared funding and other resources, including funding *specifically* to support overall cultivation and coordination of linkages.
9. Emphasis on prevention and early intervention for high-risk communities.
10. Mechanisms for providing feedback to administration regarding access, documentation of needs, and system barriers.
11. "Continuous Quality Improvement" approach emphasizing circulation of feedback, in as user-friendly a format as possible, to as many actors as possible.
12. Positions which support education and staff development and enhancements of clinical skills.
13. Flexible program design.
14. At every stage of the work—with clients, providers, and organizations—a focus on offering programs appropriate to needs and resources, and conducting them at an appropriate pace.
15. Attention to marketing and translation, to make linkage benefits clear to potential participants.

organizations, which had assumed new roles as creators, interpreters, and disseminators of new scientific information.

Meanwhile, preparing our paper on grassroots AIDS research (Indyk and Rier, 1993) sent us back to the literature on the sociology of knowledge, giving our earlier, service-driven insights a new theoretical grounding. More important, it showed us how grassroots AIDS work forces the revision and extension of dissemination theory, reinterpretations of boundaries between science and non-science, and other changes. We came to appreciate both the theoretical and political intricacies of expertise—what it is, who has it, who claims it, and why. While our service work had already shown that those without formal credentials could become knowledge producers, our theoretical analysis of grassroots AIDS research helped us to recognize that what we observed was part of a broader process with implications far beyond AIDS service and research. The next step, of course, is to extend these insights beyond the system level, and explain how the new geometry of care implies a redefinition of treatment and prevention at the individual level—for patients (Indyk & Golub). The second section of this volume extends these insights and explores the implications of the new geometry of care for patient-provider interactions.

Glaser and Strauss (1967) taught us the value of grounded research–how data must reinforce theory, and vice-versa. Our own work has involved constant interweaving of theory with praxis. It suggests a form of "grounded service": insights gleaned from service, as well as theory, should ground (or buttress) data–and vice-versa. Those who would adapt and apply the new geometry of care should be alert for similar theory-service synergies to harness to their own work.

REFERENCES

Brown, P., and Mikkelsen, E.J., 1990. *No safe place: Toxic waste, leukemia, and community action.* Berkeley: Univ. of California.

Chillag, K., Bartholow, K., Cordeiro, J., Swanson, S., Patterson, J., Stebbins, S., Woodside, C., and Sy, F., 2002. Factors affecting the delivery of HIV/AIDS prevention programs by community-based organizations. *AIDS Education and Prevention 14(3)*, 27-37.

Edelstein, M.R., 1988. *Contaminated communities: The social and psychological impacts of residential toxic exposures.* Boulder, CO: Westview.

Freidenberg J., 1991. Participatory research and grassroots development: A case study from Harlem. *City & Society 5(1)*, 64-75.

Glaser, B.G., and Strauss, A.L. (1967). *The discovery of grounded theory: Strategies for qualitative research.* NY: Aldine de Gruyter.

Indyk D., 1987. *The emergence of perinatal medicine.* Unpublished PhD dissertation, Columbia University.

Indyk, D., Belville, R., and Indyk., L. 1995. A "Total Quality Improvement" approach to community-based program development. Presented at the First International Conference on Social Work in Health and Mental Health Care. Jerusalem, January 22-26.

Indyk, D., Coury-Doniger, P., Grosz, J., Pruden, S., Jordan, S., Kaudeyr, K., Edwards, T., Klein, S., and Stevens, P.C., 1997. HIV prevention: Applying "stages of change" theory to accelerate bottom-up and top-down prevention knowledge production and technology transfer. Presented at the Public Health Conference on Records and Statistics and the National Committee on Vital and Health Statistics. Washington, D.C., July.

Indyk, D., and Indyk, L., 1995. Filling in the blanks: Creating and aggregating service-driven data to develop community profiles of special populations. pp. 398-402 in *Data Needs in an Era of Health Reform.* Proceedings of the 25th Public Health Conference on Records and Statistics and the National Committee on Vital and Health Statistics, 45th Anniversary Symposium.

Indyk, D., London, K., Tackley, L., Wennberg, J., and Heller, D., 1998. An innovative model for the provision of HIV primary care to persons otherwise lost to follow-up by traditional medical models. Presented at the XIIth International AIDS Conference [Abstract #42312]. Geneva, June 29.

Indyk, D., and Rier, D.A., 1993. Grassroots AIDS knowledge: Implications for the boundaries of science and collective action. *Knowledge: Creation, Diffusion, Utilization 15*, 3-43.

Indyk, D., and Rier, D.A., 1995. Theory-driven practice, practice-driven theory: Linking community and medical center to fight inner-city AIDS. Presented at the First International Conference on Social Work in Health and Mental Health Care. Jerusalem, January 22-26.

Indyk, D., and Rier, D.A., this volume. Wiring the HIV/AIDS system: Building interorganizational infrastructure to link people, sites, and networks. *Social Work in Health Care.*

Kegeles, S.M., Rebchook, G.M., Hays, R.B., Terry, M.A., O'Donnell, L., Leonard, N.R., Kelly, J.A., and Neumann, M.S., 2000. From science to application: The development of an intervention package. *AIDS Education and Prevention 12(Supp. A)*, 62-74.

Kraft, J.M., Mezoff, J.S., Sogolow, E.D., Neumann, M.S., and Thomas, P.A., 2000. A technology transfer model for effective HIV/AIDS interventions: Science and practice. *AIDS Education and Prevention 12(Supplement A)*, 7-20.

Kroll-Smith, S., and Floyd, H.H., 1997. *Bodies in protest: Environmental illnesses and the struggle over medical knowledge.* NY: New York University Press.

London, K., Indyk, D., Clark, J., Stancliff, S., Lee, A., Nardi, S., 1998. Results of a clinical outreach to HIV infected individuals living in SRO hotels. Presented at the XIIth International AIDS Conference [Abstract #12447]. Geneva, June 29.

McKnight, J., [1978]1990. Politicizing health care. pp. 432-436 in Conrad, P. and R. Kern (Eds.), *The sociology of health & illness* (3rd ed.). NY: St. Martin's.

Oliver, P., 1984. If you don't do it, nobody else will: Active and token contributions to local collective action. *American Journal of Sociology 49*, 601-10.

Olson, M., [1965]1971. *The logic of collective action.* Cambridge: Harvard University.

Prochaska, J.O., and DiClemente, C.C., 1986. Toward a comprehensive model of change. pp. 3-27 in W.R. Miller and N. Heather (Eds.), *Treating addictive behaviors: Processes of change.* NY: Plenum Press.

Rotheram-Borus, M.J., Rebchook. G.M., Kelly, J.A., Adams, J., and Neumann, M.S., 2000. Bridging research and practice: Community-researcher partnerships for replicating effective interventions. *AIDS Education and Prevention 12(Supplement A)*, 49-61.

Sogolow, E.D., Kay, L.S., Doll, L.S., Neumann, M.S., Mezoff, J.S., Eke, A.N., Semaan, S., and Anderson, J.R., 2000. Strengthening HIV prevention: Application of a research-to-practice framework. *AIDS Education and Prevention 12(Supp. A)*, 21-32.

Strauss, D. (this volume). A community-based organizations integration of HIV and Substance Abuse services for ex-offenders. *Social Work in Health Care.*

PART II

PATIENT-LEVEL GEOMETRY: ADHERENCE AND UNCERTAINTY– THE CHALLENGE OF PRACTICING CHANGE WHILE CHANGING PRACTICE

The Shifting Locus of Risk-Reduction: The Critical Role of HIV Infected Individuals

Debbie Indyk, PhD
Sarit A. Golub, PhD

SUMMARY. This article discusses the shifting locus of control over risk-reduction and examines its implications for the care and support of HIV-positive individuals. We begin by presenting a brief history of the continuum of HIV related risk, illustrating the ways in which advances in risk-assessment and intervention have led to this important shift. Second, we discuss the current state of risk assessment and intervention as it relates to three factors: (a) the point along the continuum of risk at which risk assessment and intervention occurs; (b) the locus of control over risk reduction; and (c) the distinction between primary and secondary risk reduction efforts. Finally, we discuss the meaning of HIV risk and the role of HIV-positive individuals in the new geometry of care that integrates treatment and prevention. How is HIV-risk defined and un-

Debbie Indyk, PhD, is affiliated with the Mount Sinai School of Medicine, New York, NY. Sarit A. Golub, PhD, is affiliated with Queens College, City University of New York.

[Haworth co-indexing entry note]: "The Shifting Locus of Risk-Reduction: The Critical Role of HIV Infected Individuals." Indyk, Debbie, and Sarit A. Golub. Co-published simultaneously in *Social Work in Health Care* (The Haworth Press, Inc.) Vol. 42, No. 3/4, 2006, pp. 113-132; and: *The Geometry of Care: Linking Resources, Research, and Community to Reduce Degrees of Separation Between HIV Treatment and Prevention* (ed: Debbie Indyk) The Haworth Press, Inc., 2006, pp. 113-132. Single or multiple copies of this article are available for a fee from The Haworth Document Delivery Service [1-800-HAWORTH, 9:00 a.m. - 5:00 p.m. (EST). E-mail address: docdelivery@haworthpress.com].

derstood? Who is of risk to whom? Who is responsible for reducing risk? *[Article copies available for a fee from The Haworth Document Delivery Service: 1-800-HAWORTH. E-mail address: <docdelivery@haworthpress.com> Website: <http://www.HaworthPress.com> © 2006 by The Haworth Press, Inc. All rights reserved.]*

KEYWORDS. Acquisition, transmission, prevention, continuum, primary and secondary risk reduction

In recent years, the notions of risk, risk assessment, and risk management have become increasingly important to the provision of health care. In part, this trend signals a shift in the way that humans are seen in relation to the health risks that surround them. Previously, health risks were seen as largely external, due to nature, genetics, or fate (asbestos exposure causes pulmonary problems; cancer runs in families). In the last decade, there has been a growing sense that many of the risks associated with disease are created and/or perpetuated by individuals (obesity and cholesterol levels associated with heart disease; smoking associated with lung cancer and emphysema). More importantly, there is a growing sense that we have the tools to eliminate or reduce these risks through medical intervention and/or health promoting behaviors. To a large extent, current medical and public health practice has shifted the "locus of control" over health risk (Skolbekken, 1995) away from external factors toward internal ones.

In order to have a meaningful discussion about reducing the risks associated with a given disease or medical problem, two conditions are necessary. First, a risk assessment tool must exist that can identify individuals at high risk of developing the disease or condition. Second, an intervention must exist that can reduce the risk. Each of these conditions is necessary but not sufficient. Consider the success of risk-reduction efforts aimed at a disease called phenylketonuria, an error of metabolism which puts newborns at risk of mental retardation. Phenylketonuria can be detected through a blood test, called a PKU, conducted immediately following birth (the risk assessment). Once detected, a special diet low in phenylalanine will allow for normal development and virtually eliminate the risk of mental retardation (the intervention). A positive PKU assessment without an understanding of the special diet intervention would be meaningless; infants would be identified as at-risk for mental retardation and their parents would simply wait and see if the risk potential was realized. Understanding of the special diet without a means to identify infants who needed it would be similarly meaningless. Therefore, meaningful risk-reduction efforts are contingent upon mastery of both risk assessment and effective interventions.

In the context of HIV infection, the concept of risk-reduction is simultaneously paramount and highly contentious. Over the past twenty-five years that we have been battling the epidemic, advances in each of the two components of successful risk reduction–assessment and intervention–have changed its meaning, and its implication for both patients and providers. The third decade of HIV requires a reassessment of treatment and prevention practices, the creation of a new "geometry of care" (Rier & Indyk, this volume). Fundamental to this new geometry of care is an understanding of the extent to which the future–and burden–of HIV risk-reduction has shifted to HIV-infected individuals.

This article discusses the shifting locus of control over risk-reduction and examines its implications for the care and support of HIV-positive individuals. We begin by presenting a brief history of the continuum of HIV related risk, illustrating the ways in which advances in risk-assessment and intervention have led to this important shift. Second, we discuss the current state of risk assessment and intervention as it relates to three factors: (a) the point along the continuum of risk at which risk assessment and intervention occurs; (b) the locus of control over risk reduction; and (c) the distinction between primary and secondary risk reduction efforts. Finally, we discuss the meaning of HIV risk and the role of HIV-positive individuals in the new geometry of care that integrates treatment and prevention. How is HIV-risk defined and understood? Who is of risk to whom? Who is responsible for reducing risk?

THE CONTINUUM OF HIV-RELATED RISK IN HISTORICAL PERSPECTIVE

The risk associated with HIV infection can be seen as a continuum, beginning when an individual is uninfected and is not engaging in any risk behaviors, and continuing through a situation in which an individual has developed AIDS and is seriously ill [Figure 1–The HIV Risk Continuum]. At each stage along the continuum, individuals are at-risk of progressing to the next stage: Uninfected individuals are at risk of infection; infected, but well individuals are at risk of disease progression; infected individuals who are seriously ill are at risk of death. At the very beginning of the AIDS epidemic, the idea of risk-reduction was not relevant, because we possessed neither reliable risk assessment tools nor

FIGURE 1. The HIV Continuum

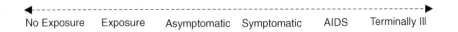

No Exposure   Exposure   Asymptomatic Symptomatic   AIDS   Terminally Ill

interventions capable of reducing risk. It was not even known that AIDS was caused by infection with a virus; individuals presented to medical centers, usually all the way at the end of the continuum, when they were already extremely ill and at risk of imminent death. There was no distinction between infected and uninfected, and no way to identify individuals "at-risk" for any of the three endpoints. Because there was no treatment for AIDS or even for many of the opportunistic infections with which infected individuals were presenting, infected individuals were faced not with the *risk* of death, but with its certainty.

The only way in which risk was discussed in the beginning of the epidemic was in the context of "risk groups," which were defined by common characteristics of the individuals who were presenting with AIDS. AIDS was known as the "4 H Club," because it was thought to occur only in *h*omosexuals, *h*eroin users, *h*emophiliacs, and *H*aitians. However, the association of AIDS with certain risk groups was not a true risk assessment; it included many members of these groups who were not at risk of infection and, as we would soon learn, excluded many individuals who were to become the future of the epidemic. In addition, a risk assessment based on membership in a "risk group" could not lead to an effective risk reduction intervention, since it was based on identity and not behavior.

As it became clear that AIDS was caused by a virus found in blood, genital secretions, and breast milk, the discussion shifted from "risk groups" to risk behaviors. The association of the disease with a virus undermined the risk continuum and divided it into two distinct stages–before infection with the virus and after infection with the virus. [Figure 2–Two Distinct Stages–Before Infection and After Infection.] In addition, this understanding formed the basis of both a tool to assess an individual's risk of infection (are you engaging in any risk behaviors?) and interventions to reduce risk (use condoms, clean needles, and/or universal precautions). A risk assessment tool was also developed to identify individuals at risk of disease progression, the HIV antibody test. However, no intervention was available to reduce the risk of progression. As a result, risk reduction efforts ignored infected individuals and focused almost exclusively on uninfected individuals engaging in high-risk behaviors [Figure 3–Early Approaches to Risk Reduction].

As knowledge about AIDS and the disease and infections associated with it grew, risk assessment and intervention efforts began to target infected individuals. Medications and treatments were developed to combat the opportunistic infections associated with AIDS and to reduce the risk of death among infected individuals [Figure 4–Risk Reduction Includes Infected Individuals]. Over the next ten years, risk reduction efforts targeting the infected and uninfected remained distinct, but were shifted earlier in the continuum. For example, risk reduction efforts targeted uninfected individuals before they began to engage in risk behaviors (for example, through school-based HIV education), and targeted infected individuals before they developed opportunistic infections (with prophylactic medications and antiretroviral therapy) [Figure 5–Shifting Focus Earlier]. However, risk-reduction efforts did not bridge populations; the dividing line separating efforts for the infected and uninfected remained absolute. The strategies for risk-reduction were also dichotomized; programs for the uninfected stressed individual behavior change, while programs for the infected relied on medical intervention.

In the mid-nineties, three intersecting advances in HIV risk assessment and intervention had tremendous implications for the meaning of HIV-related risk. First, assays were made available that allowed providers to measure an individual's "viral load"–the number of HIV RNA copies per milliliter of blood plasma. An individual's viral load is a risk assessment that has been found to be extremely predictive of progression of the illness; individuals with high levels of plasma viremia are at a greatly increased risk of clinical progression (Carpenter et al., 1998; Mellors et al., 1996). In addition to significance in its own right, the availability of viral load testing was instrumental in increasing knowledge about HIV viral dynamics–the second advance that has contributed to changes in the meaning of HIV-related risk. Research on viral dynamics has led to an understanding of the processes involved in primary infection, the first several months following contraction of the virus. Acute infection involves a tremendous increase in viral replication, in which an individual's viral load approaches or exceeds the load seen in patients with advanced AIDS (Havlir & Richman, 1996). Since the amount of HIV in blood and bodily fluids is directly related to an individual's infectiousness, primary infection is believed to account for an disproportionate amount of disease transmissions (Cates, Chesney, & Cohen, 1997; Schacker, Hughes, Shea, Coombs, & Corey, 1998). The third critical advance was the development of new, effective drugs, specifically a class of drugs known as protease inhibitors. The pairing of new medications with older antiretrovirals–called combination therapy–has been associated with a marked decrease in mortality, as well as a significant improvement in clinical symptoms (Pallela et al., 1998; Vittinghoff, Scheer, O'Malley, Colfax, Holmberg, & Buchbinder, 1999).

The intersection of these three advances had a tremendous impact on the approach to HIV treatment and management at both micro- and macro-levels. Understanding of the spike in viral levels following initial infection has led many researchers to advocate for the identification and treatment of infected individuals as early as possible (Phillips, 1996; Cates et al., 1997). Research suggests that early initiation of antiretroviral therapy may aid the individual's immune system and help maintain lower viral concentrations in both blood and semen for an extended period (Quinn, 1997; Kinloch-de Loes et al., 1995). Since there is reason to believe that early viral burden predicts long-term disease progression (Mellors, Rinaldo, Gupta, White, Todd, & Kingsley, 1996), the identification and treatment of individuals during acute infection may be critical to promoting long-term health status.

Viral load testing is an integral tool in the coordination of treatment for infected individuals, because it is a risk assessment that can be used at every point along the continuum of illness. Viral load is used as a guideline for the initiation of treatment, as a measure of treatment success, and as an indicator of the development of drug resistant strains (Powderly, Saag, Chapman, Yu, Quart, & Clendeninn, 1999). Drug resistant strains of HIV develop when the virus mutates and is able to reproduce even in the presence of medication, causing a spike in the individual's viral load. In response to such a spike, a physician may choose to change the patient's treatment regimen, in the hope that the mutated virus will be vulnerable to a different antiretroviral combination (US Department of Health and Human Services, 2005).

At the macro-level, the combination of early identification and aggressive treatment, including viral load monitoring and the adjustment of medication regimens in response to drug resistance, has transformed HIV into a chronic disease. Especially if identified early, infected individuals now live longer, healthier lives as a result of successful risk reduction efforts [Figure 6]. At the same time, the implications of these advances have had a tremendous impact on: (1) the point along the continuum of risk at which risk assessment and intervention occurs; (2) the locus of control over risk reduction; and (3) the confluence of primary and secondary risk reduction efforts.

FIGURE 2. Two Distinct Stages–Before Infection and After Infection

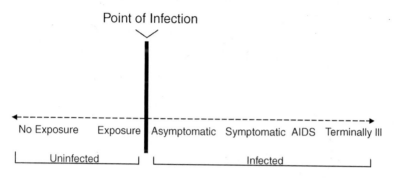

THE DISTINCTION BETWEEN PRIMARY AND SECONDARY RISK REDUCTION

Before exploring the impact on each of these three areas, it is important to understand certain terminology. In addressing the risks associated with a given disease, two terms are usually used to distinguish between intervention at different points along the continuum of illness. *Primary prevention or risk reduction* refers to efforts initiated before illness occurs that are designed to reduce the risk of developing the illness. *Secondary prevention or risk reduction* refers to efforts initiated after illness occurs that are designed to reduce the risk of further morbidity and mortality associated with the illness. For certain diseases, the interventions and programs appropriate for primary risk reduction are the same as those appropriate for secondary risk reduction. For example, similar dietary restrictions and medication regimens are recommended for both individuals with heart disease and those at high risk of developing it. However, as explained above, HIV primary and secondary risk-reduction efforts historically have been dichotomized: primary risk reduction had been restricted to uninfected individuals and has focused on individual behavior–abstinence, condom use, not sharing needles, universal precautions–while secondary risk reduction had focused on medical intervention for the infected–prophylactic medication, treatment of opportunistic infections, hospitalizations.

FIGURE 3. Early Approaches to Risk Reduction

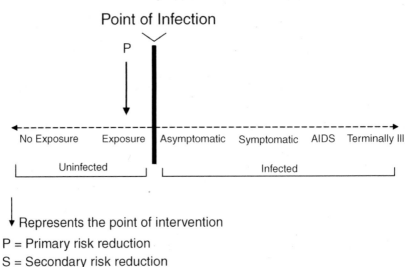

Represents the point of intervention

P = Primary risk reduction

S = Secondary risk reduction

FIGURE 4. Risk-Reduction Includes Infected Individuals

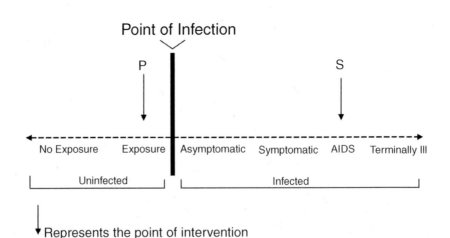

Represents the point of intervention

P = Primary risk reduction

S = Secondary risk reduction

FIGURE 5. Shifting Focus, Earlier

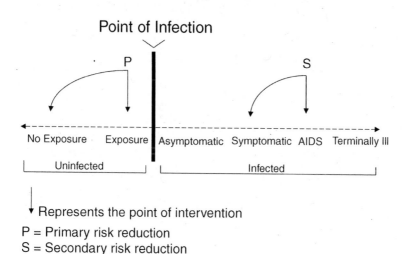

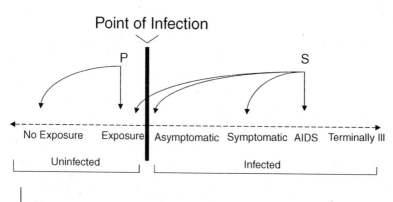

Represents the point of intervention
P = Primary risk reduction
S = Secondary risk reduction

FIGURE 6. Shifting Further Back

Represents the point of intervention
P = Primary risk reduction
S = Secondary risk reduction

LOCUS OF CONTROL OVER HIV PREVENTION AND TREATMENT

Shifting Back

Returning to the continuum of HIV-related risk, a focus on early identification and treatment shifts the locus of intervention for the infected (secondary risk reduction) to an even earlier point, almost to the moment of infection. In fact, in order to insure that HIV+ individuals are identified almost immediately after infection, secondary risk reduction efforts must also target uninfected, high-risk individuals. *Before they become infected*, high-risk individuals must be aware that effective treatments are available, must understand that these treatments are most effective when started early, must be able to recognize the symptoms of initial infection, and must know where and how to get the treatment they may need. As the point of clinical intervention and effective secondary risk reduction shifts back almost to the moment of infection, risk reduction based on medical intervention previously relevant only to the infected becomes relevant to the uninfected. In 2003, the CDC-sponsored HIV Prevention in Clinical Care Working Group published recommendations for incorporating HIV prevention into the medical care of individuals living with HIV (CDC, 2003). These recommendations acknowledge the extent to which risk-assessment of behaviors and clinical factors associated with transmission of HIV and other Sexually Transmitted Infections (STIs) can be used to identify HIV-positive patients who are in need of risk-reduction counseling and/or other interventions [Figure 7–Shifting Further Back].

A New Locus

As noted above, over the past several decades the locus of control of risk has shifted from nature to humans and now resides in medical knowledge and intervention (Skolbekken, 1995). The implications of recent advances in HIV assessment and intervention have shifted the locus of control over risk even further, from medical providers to patients themselves. Management of HIV as a chronic illness requires medical expertise and supervision, but its success is dependent upon the consistent action of HIV-infected individuals themselves. The majority of drug treatments for HIV, including protease inhibitors, work by destroying the virus' ability to replicate itself (Hammer, 1996). As mentioned above, the virus is sometimes able to mutate, creating a viral type

FIGURE 7. Shifting Back and Forward

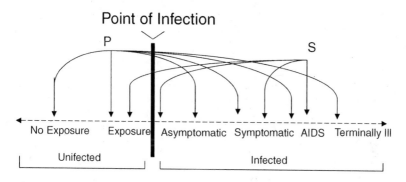

Point of Infection

↓ Represents the point of intervention

P = Primary risk reduction

S = Secondary risk reduction

that can reproduce even in the presence of the drug. The likelihood of viral mutation increases if individuals do not adhere precisely to their prescribed treatment regimen. An increase in a patient's viral load is a good indicator of such a mutation and often suggests a need for an adjustment of the treatment regimen in the hope that a different combination will be effective in keeping viral titers low. If a patient's viral load is not checked regularly, a viral mutation might be allowed to reproduce to a level that would not be controlled by changing drug combinations. Therefore, in order to reduce the risk of drug failure, infected individuals must: (1) adhere precisely to medication regimens in terms of timing and dosage; and (2) visit their physician on a regular basis in order to monitor their viral load. In the case of drug failure due to insufficient monitoring of viral load or non-adherence to treatment regimens, an individual could be infected with a drug-resistant strain of the virus and be unable to take advantage of any of the treatments currently available.

In addition, if HIV is to be managed as a chronic illness, basic health promotion activities become extremely important to infected individuals. While the immune systems of infected individuals are strengthened by drug treatment, they are still more vulnerable to infections and illnesses which could compromise their health. In addition, coinfection with other diseases can accelerate progression of HIV itself and can reduce the effectiveness of combination therapy. For example, Hepatitis C can be lethal in individuals who are immuno-compromised (Rockstrojh et al.,

1996). In addition, since drug therapies put a strain on the liver, individuals with liver damage as a result of hepatitis infection may be unable to tolerate necessary medication regimens. In another example, researchers have demonstrated higher rates of invasive cervical cancer (ICC) among HIV-positive women; in one study, HIV-infected women's prevalence of dysplasia/neoplasia was ten times that of a control outpatient population and four times that of a control population of HIV-negative intravenous drug users (Shafer et al., 1992). A large body of evidence suggests that cervical cancer is caused by a sexually transmitted disease called Human Papilloma virus (HPV) and that the aggressive progression of neoplasia is related to the degree of a woman's immunosuppression (Bowman & Spangler, 1995).

Therefore, as HIV emerges as a chronic disease, effective secondary risk reduction depends on infected individuals' adopting a series of health promoting behaviors. Acute disease is usually treated within a hospital or other medical facility where medications are administered and procedures are performed with the patient as a passive recipient. The management of a chronic illness must take place outside the medical center, within the context of the patient's everyday life. Patients must become active participants in their treatment plans; taking medications and engaging in other health maintenance behaviors. Therefore, the advances that make it possible for HIV+ individuals to live longer, healthier lives also shift the locus of secondary risk reduction. As the focus of effective risk reduction becomes individual behavior, the locus of risk reduction shifts from medical providers to infected individuals themselves. Of course, secondary risk reduction cannot take place without medical care and supervision; however, the focus must be on a *partnership* between medical providers and their patients. As the new geometry of care recognizes the role of HIV-infected individuals in knowledge-production and the development of new expertise, the shifting locus of control over HIV-risk reduction recognizes the role of HIV-infected individuals in enacting treatment and prevention goals.

Shifting Forward

Unfortunately, the behaviors on which successful secondary risk reduction now relies are often difficult and unpleasant. Adherence to medication regimens is a complicated and arduous process. While recent advances in the pharmaceutical industry have greatly simplified the timing and burden of drug treatment regimens, the burden of adherence is still borne by HIV-positive individuals (see Golub & Indyk, this volume; O'Brien, Clark, Besch, Myers, & Kissinger, 2003). Many of the medications have unpleasant side effects, ranging from nausea and dizziness to kidney damage and hearing loss (Fellay et al., 2001) Frequent trips to the doctor can also be difficult for infected individuals who are living healthier lives that include jobs and parenting. Many infected individuals are battling drug addiction which can affect their ability to follow regimens and keep scheduled appointments.

The health maintenance behaviors that help individuals avoid coinfections are also extremely difficult. While this health maintenance regimen includes general behaviors like a balanced diet and adequate rest, it also includes behaviors usually associated with primary risk reduction–using condoms, clean needles, and universal precautions. Hepatitis C is endemic among injection drug users (Wright et al., 1994), making the adoption of safer needle-using practices critical for HIV+ injection drug users. Human Papilloma Virus is just one of many sexually transmitted diseases that should be avoided by infected individuals in order to maintain their health status, making safer sex critical for HIV+ individuals who are sexually active.

Therefore, while traditional secondary risk reduction efforts must be shifted *back* to include uninfected individuals, traditional primary risk reduction efforts must be shifted *forward* to include infected individuals. In the past, one of the reasons that HIV+ individuals were not targeted by primary prevention programs was the argument that infected individuals had no motivation to use condoms or clean needles. The success of triple combination therapy has created such incentives. As HIV+ individuals are faced with the prospect of living longer, healthier lives, risk reduction for the uninfected becomes relevant to the infected. Primary risk reduction strategies are now crucial components of secondary prevention efforts [Figure 7–Shifting Back and Forward].

THE CONFLUENCE OF PRIMARY
AND SECONDARY RISK REDUCTION

As similar risk reduction behaviors and activities become relevant to both infected and uninfected individuals, the line between primary and secondary risk reduction begins to blur. In fact, when HIV-positive individuals engage in secondary risk reduction behaviors, these behaviors act simultaneously as primary risk reduction for uninfected individuals. For example, in order to reduce their risk of coinfection with sexually transmitted diseases or other blood borne pathogens that might exacerbate their illness, HIV-infected individuals may choose to use condoms consistently or refrain from sharing needles. For infected individuals, these behaviors are a form of *secondary* risk reduction, because they are designed to reduce the risk of further morbidity and mortality associated with HIV. However, for their sexual or needle sharing partners who are HIV-negative, these actions become effective means of *primary* risk reduction; safer sexual and/or needle sharing practices reduce the risk of HIV transmission from infected to uninfected partners. Therefore, targeting HIV-positive individuals with information and education regarding risk-reduction practices that were traditionally thought of as relevant only to uninfected individuals (abstaining from risky behaviors, reducing the number of sexual partners, using condoms and other latex barriers, not sharing needles, cleaning needles with bleach) is now at the same time, an effective method of primary *and* secondary prevention.

Similarly, when infected individuals check their viral load regularly and adhere to drug treatment regimens they are engaging in *secondary* risk reduction, since these behaviors reduce their risk of developing drug resistant strains of the virus that would lead to disease progression. But reducing the risk of the development of drug resistant strains of HIV can also be seen as a form of *primary* risk reduction, because it reduces the risk that this drug resistant virus will be transmitted to uninfected individuals. In addition, research suggests that individuals with lower viral load are less infectious to others, since they have a lower concentration of virus in their blood stream and bodily fluids (Baeten & Overbaugh, 2003). For this reason, secondary risk reduction practices that reduce the infected individual's viral load become effective means of primary risk reduction, because, by reducing the infectiousness of infected individuals, they reduce the risk of HIV transmission to uninfected individuals.

Therefore, HIV-positive individuals are critical in preventing transmission to uninfected individuals. If all infected individuals were vigilant about secondary risk reduction behaviors–including regular monitoring of viral load, adherence to drug treatment regimens, consistent condom use, and abstinence from needle sharing–the spread of HIV infection would be greatly reduced, *even if uninfected individuals did not engage in primary risk reduction*. This is not to suggest that primary risk reduction efforts should not target the uninfected; rather, it underscores the critical role of HIV-positive individuals in both the continued success of early treatment efforts and in the management of disease transmission.

Perhaps the most striking example of the confluence of primary and secondary risk reduction in the actions of infected individuals has been the use of zidovudine (commonly called AZT or ZDV) therapy during pregnancy to prevention transmission from mother to fetus. In 1994, a clinical trial found that the use of ZDV during pregnancy, labor, and the months immediately following birth decreased the likelihood of perinatal transmission from 25% to 8% (Conner et al., 1994). Since that time, guidelines for reducing maternal-child transmission recommend that all HIV-positive pregnant women receive antiretroviral therapy (US Department of Health and Human Services, 2005). Since drug therapy can also improve outcomes for the infected individuals, HIV-positive pregnant women who take ZDV during pregnancy are engaging in primary and secondary risk reduction *simultaneously*; they are reducing the risk of transmission to the fetus (primary risk reduction) and reducing the risk of progression of their own illness (secondary risk reduction). In the case of perinatal transmission, the locus of primary risk reduction rests exclusively on the infected individual, since the uninfected fetus is unable to participate in risk reduction. Perinatal transmission also underscores the dual forces that may motivate the adoption of risk reduction behavior–altruism and self-interest.[1]

As mentioned above, it was often argued that HIV-positive individuals had no reason to engage in risk reduction behavior because of their impending illness and death. While certain authors maintained that aggressive counseling and testing would lower the incidence of transmission by encouraging infected individuals to modify their behavior, studies found a weak correlation between knowledge of one's status and adoption of risk reduction practices. This fueled the argument that altruism was not a good motivator of behavior change and contributed to the separation of programs for the infected and uninfected. The fact that the same behaviors represent both primary and secondary risk reduction means that the same behaviors can be motivated by altruism and self-interest. Infected individuals now have a self-interest in risk reduction behaviors that are also inherently altruistic.

ORGANIZATIONAL SHIFTS AND THE LOCATION OF HIV-RELATED RISK WITHIN SOCIETY

An effective response to the changes discussed above requires a shift in the organization and delivery of HIV-related services and a reevaluation of the placement of HIV-related risk within society. First, the current system of HIV care and prevention is not equipped to handle the shift in focus of risk reduction efforts and the blurring of the distinction between primary and secondary risk reduction. In addition to being dichotomized in their population base (infected vs. uninfected individuals), secondary and primary prevention have also been dichotomized in terms of funding, training, and structures. As mentioned above, the creation of new interventions represents a shift in emphasis from secondary risk reduction driven by a medical model (administration of medication and procedures) to secondary risk reduction driven by a behavioral model (adherence to treatment and transmission prevention practices). Primary risk reduction interventions must begin to incorporate treatment education and updates and must strengthen their ties to testing centers and medical facilities.

Second, the current system of HIV care and prevention is not equipped to handle the shift in the locus of risk reduction efforts toward a partnership between medical providers and infected individuals. Collaboration between providers and patients is not the norm, and most treatment facilities do not have programs that support and encourage adherence to treatment regimens and risk reduction related to sexual behavior and needle use. However, the creation, assessment, and replication of client-centered risk reduction requires such collaboration. Both of these shifts—integrating primary and secondary prevention and increasing collaboration between providers and patients—are integral to the new geometry of care for HIV. Many of the systemic and organizational-level changes needed to support these shifts are discussed in the articles in this volume's first section.

Third, a reevaluation of the role of the infected individual in effecting risk reduction goals leads to a reevaluation of the placement of risk within society. While we have discussed the shifts inherent in HIV becoming a chronic disease, it continues to be infectious, thus raising public health concerns associated with infectious disease. Infectious disease is simultaneously a risk to individuals and a risk to society as a whole. The behaviors associated with infectious disease can be behaviors that put individuals themselves at risk or behaviors that put others at risk.

In the case of most infectious diseases, once an individual has contracted the disease, engaging in behaviors that can transmit the disease may put *others* at risk, but present no further risk to the index case. For example, once an individual has contracted tuberculosis, being in an enclosed, poorly ventilated room with other people presents a risk only to the uninfected. There may be other behaviors that put the infected individual at risk of increased severity of the illness (like walking around in the rain with no coat), but an individual with an infectious disease is primarily a risk to society. This paradigm applied to HIV when the epidemic first began. Once an individual was infected, it was believed that engaging in traditional risky behaviors was no longer a threat to her health. HIV+ individuals were seen primarily as a risk to society.

There have been many different approaches to controlling individuals who present risks to society (quarantine, directly observed therapy); however, most of them have been punitive and have centered around separating infected individuals from the rest of society. Similar measures were considered to control the HIV epidemic; the proposals included quarantine of infected individuals and mandatory testing.

Now that the same behaviors that pose a risk to society also pose a risk to the HIV-infected person himself, the risk reduction methodology adopted must insure a collaboration, not separation, between infected individuals and society. However, if the need to target risk reduction to those who are already infected is seen as a public health need to reduce collective risk, then there are those who would choose a methodology that is both punitive and stigmatizing. There is a danger that the shift in locus of control and the confluence of primary and secondary risk reduction goals could lead to a shift of primary responsibility to infected individuals to prevent the epidemic. This paper is not suggesting that we shift the responsibility away from societal responsibility to the individual. Rather, we advocate a shift in the locus of support toward a partnership between the infected and the uninfected. As HIV becomes a chronic illness, infected individuals must live within society, not outside it. As such, the responsibility of reducing risk for both individuals and society must reside with society as a whole. As we shape the future of HIV care and prevention, there is an imperative to create interventions that reduce collective risk by supporting individuals.

However, this shift cannot be undertaken without a fundamental increase in understanding of the realities of the lives of HIV-infected individuals. One of the clearest intersections and interactions between HIV-positive individuals and their providers is around the issue of treatment adherence. If we are to truly support HIV-infected individuals as a new locus of control, we must understand treatment adherence within the context of the complex, often competing demands of living with a chronic illness. This section of this volume presents a series of articles that move this discussion forward, presenting different approaches to understanding and supporting treatment adherence. HIV-positive individuals represent a new locus of control for both traditionally population-based public health measures and client-level interventions; integrating these into the new geometry of care requires the convergence of prevention and treatment into a continuum of care.

NOTE

1. It is important to note that antiretroviral therapy is recommended for pregnant women, regardless of whether or not the woman has chosen to initiate treatment for her own disease. In some cases, preventing maternal-child transmission might entail a change of regimen for the mother, and might expose her to the possibility of increased side effects, toxicity, or even future drug-resistant virus (Lyons et al., 2002). As a result, the best interests of the mother and her fetus do not always coincide, and initiation of drug therapy to prevent maternal-child transmission must be done in the context of a comprehensive risk-benefit analysis.

REFERENCES

Baeten, J.M., & Overbaugh, J. (2003). Measuring the infectiousness of persons with HIV-1: opportunities for preventing sexual HIV-1 transmission. *Current HIV Research, 1*(1), 69-86.

Bowman, M.A,. & Spangler J.G. (1995). Screening, health promotion, and prevention in women. *Primary Care, 22*(4), 661-77.

Cardo, D.M., Culver, D.H., Ciesielski, C.A. et al. (1997). A case-control study of HIV seroconversion in health care workers after percutaneous exposure. *New England Journal of Medicine, 337,* 1485–90.

Carpenter, C.C., Fischl, M.A., Hammer, S.M., Hirsch, M.S., Jacobsen, D.M., Katzenstein, D.A., Montaner, J.S., Richman, D.D., Saag, M.S., Schooley, R.T., Thompson, M.A., Vella, S., Yeni, P.G., Volberding, P.A. (1998). Antiretroviral Therapy for HIV Infection in 1996: Recommendations of an International Panel. *Journal of the American Medical Association, 280*(1), 78-86.

Cates, W. Jr., Chesney, M.A., & Cohen, M.S. (1997). Primary HIV infection–A public health opportunity. *American Journal of Public Health, 87*(12), 1928-1930.

Centers for Disease Control and Prevention. (1995). Case-control Study of HIV Seroconversion in Health-Care Workers after Percutaneous Exposure to HIV-infected Blood–France, United Kingdom, and United States, January 1988-August 1994. *MMWR Morbidity and Mortality Weekly Report, 44,* 929-933.

Centers for Disease Control and Prevention (2003). Incorporating HIV prevention into the medical care of persons living with HIV: Recommendations of CDC, the Health Resources and Services Administration, the National Institutes of Health, and the HIV Medicine Association of the Infectious Diseases Society of America. *MMWR Morbidity and Mortality Weekly Report, 52*(RR-12), 1-24.

Centers for Disease Control and Prevention (2005). Antiretroviral postexposure prophylaxis after sexual, injection-drug use, or other nonoccupational exposure to HIV in the United States. *MMWR Morbidity and Mortality Weekly Report, 54*(RR01), 1-20.

Conner, E.M., Sperling, R.S., Gelber, R., Kiselev, P., Scott, G., O'Sullivan, M.J., VanDyke, R., Bey, M., Shearer, W., Jacobson, R.L. et al. (1994). Reduction of maternal-infant transmission of human immunodeficiency virus type 1 with zidovudine treatment. *New England Journal of Medicine, 331,* 1173-1180.

Dragoni, F., Mazzucconi, M.G., Cafolla, A. et al. (1996). Rapid liver failure related to chronic C hepatitis in a HIV seropositive hemophilic patient with severe immuno-depression. *Haematologica, 81*(4):335-8.

Fellay, J., Boubaker, K., Ledergerber, B., Bernasconi, E., Furrer, H., Battegay, M., Hirschel, B., Vernazza, P., Francioli, P., Greub, G., Flepp, M., Telenti, A. & the Swiss HIV Cohort Study. (2001). Prevalence of adverse events associated with potent antiretroviral treatment: Swiss HIV Cohort Study. *Lancet, 358*(9290), 1322-1327.

Hammer, S.M. (1996). Advances in antiretroviral therapy and viral load monitoring. *AIDS, 10*(Suppl 3): S1-11.

Havlir, D.V. & Richman, D.D. (1996). Viral dynamics of HIV: Implications for drug development and therapeutic strategies. *Annals of Internal Medicine, 124*(11), 984-994.

Kinloch-de Loes, S., Hirschel, B.J., Hoen, B. (1995). A controlled trial of zidovudine in primary human immunodeficiency virus infection. *New England Journal of Medicine, 333*, 408-413.

Lyons, F., Coughlan, S., Byrne, C. et al. (2002). Emergence of genotypic resistance in HIV-1-infected pregnant taking HAART to reduce mother-to-child transmission of HIV-1. 11th Conference on Retroviruses and Opportunistic Infections. San Francisco, CA, February 24-28, (Abstract 892).

Mellors, J.W., Kingsley, L.A., Rinaldo, C.R. Jr., Todd, J.A., Hoo, B.S., Kokka, R.P., & Gupta, P. (1995). Quantitation of HIV-1 RNA in plasma predicts outcome after seroconversion. *Annals of Internal Medicine, 122*:573-9.

Mellors, J.W., Rinaldo, C.R. Jr., Gupta, P., White, R.M., Todd, J.A., Kingsley, L.A. (1996) Prognosis in HIV-1 infection predicted by the quantity of virus in plasma. *Science, 272*, 1167-1170.

O'Brien, M.E., Clark, R.A., Besch, C.L., Myers, L., & Kissinger, P. (2003). Patterns and correlates of discontinuation of the initial HAART regimen in an urban outpatient cohort. *Journal of Acquired Immune Deficiency Syndrome, 34*(4), 407-14.

Palella, F.J., Jr., Delaney, K.M., Moorman, A.C., Loveless, M.O., Fuhrer, J., Satten, G.A., Aschman, D.J., & Holmberg, S.D. (1998). Declining morbidity and mortality among patients with advanced human immunodeficiency virus infection. *Journal of the American Medical Association, 338*(13), 853-60.

Phillips, A.N. (1996). Reduction of HIV Concentration During Acute Infection: Independence from a Specific Immune Response. *Science, 271*, 497-499.

Powderly, W.G., Saag, M.S., Chapman, S., Yu, G., Quart, B., & Clendeninn, N.J. (1999). Predictors of optimal virological response to potent antiretroviral therapy. *AIDS, 13*(14), 1873-1880

Quinn, T.A. (1997). Acute primary HIV infection. *Journal of the American Medical Association, 278*, 58-62.

Rockstrojh, J.K., Spengler U., Sudhop, T. et al. (1996). "Immunosuppression May Lead to Progression of Hepatitis C Virus-associated Liver Disease in Hemophiliacs Coinfected with HIV. *American Journal of Gastroenterology, 91*(12): 2563-8.

Schacker, T.W., Hughes, J.P., Shea, T., Coombs, R.W., & Corey, L. (1998). Biological and virologic characteristics of primary HIV infection. *Annals of Internal Medicine, 128*(8), 613-620.

Shafer, A., Friedmann, W., Mielke, M., Schafer, A., Schwartlander, B., & Koch, M.A. (1991). The increased frequency of cervical dysplasia-neoplasia in women infected with the Human Immunodeficiency Virus is related to the degree of immunosuppression. *American Journal of Obstetrics and Gynecology, 164*:593.

Skolbekken J.A. (1995). The risk epidemic in medical journals. *Social Science in Medicine, 40*(3):291-305.

US Department of Health And Human Services (2005). Guidelines for the use of antiretroviral agents in HIV-1-infected adults and adolescents. April, 2005. Available at: *http://aidsinfo.nih.gov/guidelines/adult/AA_040705.pdf*

Vittinghoff, E., Scheer, S., O'Malley, P., Colfax, G., Holmberg, S.D., & Buchbinder, S.P. (1999). Combination antiretroviral therapy and recent declines in AIDS incidence and mortality. *Journal of Infectious Diseases, 179*(3), 717-720.

Wright, T.L., Hollander, H., Pu, X., Held, M.J., Lipson, P., Quan, S., Polito, A., Thaler, M.M., Bacchetti, P., & Scharschmidt, B.F. (1994). Hepatitis C in HIV-infected patients with and without AIDS: Prevalence and relationship to patient survival. *Hepatology, 20*(5), 1152-1155.

Flexible Rigidity:
Supporting HIV Treatment Adherence in a Rapidly-Changing Treatment Environment

David A. Rier, PhD
Debbie Indyk, PhD

SUMMARY. This paper examines adherence to AIDS treatment, focusing on the challenges posed by rapidly changing treatment protocols. We examine the evolving views of treatment adherence, and endorse the "concordance" approach. This emphasizes collaboration and negotiation between provider and patient to formulate and maintain a manageable treatment regimen tailored to what the patient is ready, willing, and able to tolerate. Given the extreme rapidity with which treatment guidelines are revised or even reversed, the persistent uncertainty surrounding treatment risks and benefits, and the great variability in individuals' ability to tolerate a given regimen, we propose the term "flexible rigidity" to describe the type of adherence best suited to AIDS treatment. We present an organizational approach to supporting the type of provider-patient relationships needed to improve treatment adherence that features treatment-readiness assessment and custom-tailoring of treatment for those

David A. Rier, PhD, is affiliated with Bar-Ilan University, Ramat-Gan, Israel. Debbie Indyk, PhD, is affiliated with the Mount Sinai School of Medicine, New York, NY.

[Haworth co-indexing entry note]: "Flexible Rigidity: Supporting HIV Treatment Adherence in a Rapidly-Changing Treatment Environment." Rier, David A., and Debbie Indyk. Co-published simultaneously in *Social Work in Health Care* (The Haworth Press, Inc.) Vol. 42, No. 3/4, 2006, pp. 133-150; and: *The Geometry of Care: Linking Resources, Research, and Community to Reduce Degrees of Separation Between HIV Treatment and Prevention* (ed: Debbie Indyk) The Haworth Press, Inc., 2006, pp. 133-150. Single or multiple copies of this article are available for a fee from The Haworth Document Delivery Service [1-800-HAWORTH, 9:00 a.m. - 5:00 p.m. (EST). E-mail address: docdelivery@haworthpress.com].

at *all* stages of the treatment-readiness continuum. We note that this model could be applied as well to prevention and management of other chronic diseases. *[Article copies available for a fee from The Haworth Document Delivery Service: 1-800-HAWORTH. E-mail address: <docdelivery@haworthpress.com> Website: <http://www.HaworthPress.com> © 2006 by The Haworth Press, Inc. All rights reserved.]*

KEYWORDS. AIDS treatment, adherence, concordance, chronic illness, clinical treatment guidelines

The AIDS epidemic has redefined relations between science and citizen, between doctor and patient. This paper explores a particular facet of one such change: the changing doctor-patient dynamic regarding patient adherence to medical regimens. In earlier work, we explored how actors at all locations in the system (academic researchers, patients, clinicians, community-based service providers) have unique expertise that must be harnessed (Rier and Indyk, this volume), and described our service model of multi-level linkages through which these expertise can be tapped (Indyk and Rier, this volume).

In the present paper, we apply these insights to the following question: What type of service design best supports AIDS treatment adherence when both doctors and patients struggle with rapidly-shifting treatment protocols? After an overview of how the concept of patient adherence has evolved over recent decades, we discuss the significance, for doctors and patients, of the fact that AIDS treatment guidelines and practices change very quickly. We next examine, via a look at one innovative adherence model, the features of service design and delivery necessary to support the newly evolving doctor-patient relationship. Finally, we briefly consider how these principles apply to prevention and management of other chronic diseases.

The arrival of the HAART (highly active antiretroviral therapy) treatment in the mid-1990s brought new hope to HIV+/AIDS patients, and rapidly, markedly, lowered AIDS morbidity and mortality rates where it was widely used (Palella, Delaney, Moorman, Loveless, Fuhrer et al., 1998). Nevertheless, patient compliance with this potentially life-saving treatment has been problematic. Actually, patient non-compliance with treatment is one of the better-documented facts in medicine, with rates typically reported at the 50% level (Sackett and Snow, 1979; Donovan and Blake, 1992). The problem is global. A World Health Organization

(WHO) report recently declared that, in developed nations, long-term adherence to chronic disease treatments averaged 50%, while in developing nations the rates are still lower (WHO, 2003:xiii). Though significant adherence problems exist across the range of chronic illnesses (Carter, Taylor, and Levenson, 2003), the problem is particularly serious with AIDS. Not only is the disease lethal, but current clinical thinking holds that adherence must be extremely high (as high as 95%) in order to manage HIV infection and prevent development of drug-resistant strains–which can then be transmitted to others (Chesney, 2003; Chesney, Morrin, and Sher, 2000). Indeed, adherence may be *the* critical factor in managing HIV/AIDS (WHO, 2003, pg. 101).

Accordingly, much research has focused on the problem of non-adherence to HAART (Chesney, 2003; Remien, Hirky, Johnson, Weinhardt, Whittier, and Le, 2003; Van Servellen, Chang, Garcia, and Lombardi, 2002). Research has often sought to identify key obstacles to patient compliance. Factors which have been identified include: the often-severe, highly unpleasant side-effects; the high cost of treatment; psychological factors; and problems with the structure of medical care and health service delivery.

The adherence obstacle receiving perhaps the most attention has been the complexity of the drug regimen: the number and variety of pills, the number of times a day these must be consumed, requirements to take them on an empty or full stomach, etc. Over time, there have been improvements in this area, as simpler regimens have been developed. Yet such changes, however welcome, involve their own difficulties.

For these changes can contribute a subtle obstacle to treatment compliance, one that has received far less notice: the difficulty that professionals have in driving home the "adherence message" when the *content* of that message shifts faster than it does for most other kinds of treatment. This paper addresses this problem as it applies to HAART adherence. We discuss what it implies about how doctors and patients must work together to achieve treatment goals not just for AIDS, but for other diseases as well. We explore the implications for service design and delivery appropriate to an era in which treatments are rapidly evolving, and involve negotiations between patients and doctors.

From Compliance to Adherence, From Adherence to Concordance

How we think about patient compliance has shifted with time. As observers from Zola (1987[1981]) to Brittten (2001) have noted, non-compliance was originally regarded as a failure on the part of the patient, whether through laziness, fear, ignorance, etc., to heed the physician's instructions. "Non-compliant" patients have been tagged with various harsh, stigmatizing labels over the years (Lerner, Gulick, and Dubler, 1998; Steiner and Earnest, 2000).

However, subsequent research began to revise this view (Steiner and Earnest, 2000). Zola (1987[1981]), himself, pointed to problems in doctor-communication as contributing to patients' poor compliance. He noted the various asymmetries in the doctor-patient relationship that could stifle communication and collaboration, and described how harried physicians often failed to devote the time necessary to explain the treatment and its implications. As a result, patients were often left unsure of how, exactly, they were meant to take the medication, and unprepared to face its possible side-effects. Such analyses by Zola and others (e.g., Svarstad, 1976; Hulka, 1979) reflected an important change, since they more evenly distributed responsibility for compliance problems. Indeed, Zola called for physicians to ally themselves with patients, to negotiate, together, the path to improved treatments experiences.

Additional insights emerged from Conrad's (1985) study of epilepsy patients, which focused on how the patients themselves viewed medications. Conrad questioned the whole concept of compliance. He highlighted its latent assumption that what the physician prescribed was necessarily correct, and that any patient departure from these instructions therefore necessarily constituted deviant behavior to be controlled. He pointed out how little patients' compliance practices actually had to do with physicians and the doctor-patient relationship. Instead, Conrad (extending earlier work by social psychologists such as Becker, Maiman, Kirscht et al., 1979) observed that patients made medication decisions according to what matched their daily lives, goals, and priorities. Another important finding was the extent to which patients *self-regulated* medication. Often they raised, lowered, or intermittently stopped medication in a bid to find the combination that worked best for them, and, also, to assert a degree of control over the disease's hold on their lives.

Subsequent studies (e.g., Donovan and Blake, 1992; Townsend, Hunt, and Wyke, 2003) have confirmed and extended this by pointing out that, though there is indeed much experimentation and non-compliance with doctors' instructions, this is often the product of patients' logical cost-benefit analyses, rather than fear, laziness, inability to comprehend, etc. Indeed, that non-adherence to protocols may sometimes be not only reasonable but appropriate has also been noted in other fields, such as in the aviation safety literature (Karwal, Verkaik, and Jansen, 2000).

Such insights have pointed to the complexity of the compliance issue, and have led to a view of patients as active agents in their own treatment, rather than merely passive objects of the physician's ministrations. As such, it has become more common to conceptualize treatment as a process in which physicians and patients work together to negotiate the optimum experience (Lerner, Gulick, and Dubler, 1998).

This change has been reflected in evolving nomenclature. In the 1990s, the term "adherence," which was thought to bear less authoritarian connotations, gained favor as an alternative to "compliance," and is currently the standard term in use. Participants at a 2001 WHO meeting started by defining adherence, in a way quite close to the traditional concept of "compliance," as the extent to which patients follow medical instructions. However, they felt that the term "instructions" inappropriately portrayed the patient as a "passive, acquiescent recipient of expert advice," rather than as "active collaborator" in treatment (cited in WHO, 2003:3). Noting the importance of a patient-provider partnership that allows for negotiation, the conference participants in the end adopted the following definition: "the extent to which a person's behavior . . . corresponds with agreed recommendations from a health care provider" (quoted in WHO, 2003:3).

With this, the concept of adherence converged with another term, "concordance." By 1997, a joint working party of the Royal Pharmaceutical Society of Great Britain and drug maker Merck, Sharpe, and Dohme had explicitly embraced the notion of therapeutic alliance that was earlier articulated by Zola, and that was consistent with Conrad's view of patients' medication practices as reflecting their legitimate reckonings. This was embodied in a new concept, concordance, intended to replace compliance and adherence:

> The pursuit of "compliance" has hitherto suggested that the aim of prescribing was to get the patient "to follow doctor's orders." There was an unspoken assumption that the patient's role was to be passive and that since the prescriber's view was rational and evidence-based, it was, for these reasons, "superior" to the beliefs and wishes of the patient. . . . Concordance is based on the notion that the work of prescriber and patient in the consultation is a negotiation between equals and that therefore the aim is a therapeutic alliance between them. . . . Its strength lies in a new assumption of respect for the patient's agenda and the creation of openness in the

relationship, so that both doctor and patient together can proceed on the basis of reality and not of misunderstanding, distrust or concealment. (Working Party, 1997, p. 8)

Commenting on concordance, Weiss and Britten (2003) remarked that a key way in which this model differed from that of compliance was in its promoting power sharing between provider and patient, and in respecting the patient's perspective. Rather than constituting a paternalistic, top-down model, concordance acknowledges (and taps) patients' unique expertise regarding their own body's experiences of, and reactions to, treatment. As we will see, such a concept may be particularly suited for the types of patient medication behaviors, physician prescribing practices, and indeed, the state of biomedical knowledge, found in our contemporary experience with the AIDS epidemic.

THE FLUID NATURE OF AIDS TREATMENT PROTOCOL AND PRACTICES

When discussing compliance or adherence to the drug regimen that a physician prescribes, there usually exists an assumption (if often unstated) that solid clinical research supports the physician's treatment plan. It is understood that changing knowledge may well lead to refinements, or even significant changes in treatment protocols (and, of course, physicians will often tinker with recommended dosages, etc., in an effort to strike the right balance between efficacy and side effects), but substantial changes are generally few and far between, since the development and articulation of a professional consensus often takes years. Typically, the process goes something like this: First, a body of clinical trials must be designed, funded, and conducted. Preliminary results are often presented and sometimes debated at scientific conferences, which stage is then followed by journal publication. Once a group of studies has accumulated, professional societies, government agencies, and other bodies may, if the matter is important enough, convene to seek a consensus on appropriate treatment standards. If consensus is reached, then recommended treatment protocols–the ultimate fruits of a process involving years of labor–may be formulated to serve as clinical guidelines for the coming years. These protocols must be disseminated, traditionally through professional publications and then through clinical "opinion leaders," and finally down to the rank-and-file physicians in the trenches, many of whom never really get the word or fully assimilate its message.

With AIDS, this scenario has played out differently. Several factors have combined to produce a vastly accelerated, and truncated process of altering treatment practices that is redefining the very nature of treatment protocols. First, since AIDS is a new disease, and the current HAART treatment is newer still, there has not yet been the time to build a stable therapeutic knowledge base, as there has been for most forms of cancer or heart disease. Thus, drug combinations and dosages are often very much a matter of trial and error by physicians and patients. Second, the severity of AIDS, combined with the power and organization of HIV/AIDS patient activism, has placed immense pressure on the system to bring new treatments into clinical use ("drugs into bodies," as the slogan went), thus substantially shortening the time during which these drugs are tested. As one participant in the process of formulating treatment guidelines observed:

> AIDS activists have been phenomenally successful: HIV medications are approved faster than any other drugs, and protease inhibitors were approved faster than any drugs in history. But that success is a mixed blessing. Drugs get out of the pipeline faster, but with less data about how to use them properly. And once the drugs hit the market, it becomes harder to do the randomized, controlled studies necessary to find out how best to use them. (Barr, 2000)

Moreover, instead of the structured dissemination process typical of other disease treatments, here there is intense, focused interest on the part of researchers, clinicians–and also patients, who often learn of new treatment protocols as soon as they are announced, via Internet.

Two features of the AIDS treatment scene stand out for our present discussion. First, dissemination is no longer strictly top-down: Patients do not necessarily learn of new treatments or treatment combinations directly through their physician. Apart from the traditional grapevine of friends and co-workers, etc., there exists an elaborate network of Internet chat-rooms, mailing lists, and support groups. These supplement, and sometimes are the direct online descendants of, the printed activist newsletters and other AIDS information dissemination devices that arose during the 1980s and both reflected–and constituted–a social movement that challenged traditional hierarchical dissemination patterns (Indyk and Rier, 1993). Such channels promote dissemination and assessment of bulletins from the medical world, while also enabling those living with HIV/AIDS to exchange insights and suggestions with one another about managing side effects, varying medication doses, or even intermittently stopping medication.

Not all those affected–particularly in the inner city–engage in such Internet activities. Yet enough do, as to suggest that this degree of innovation and experimentation amounts nearly to a *communal* form of the self-regulation that Conrad (1985) noted. In such a climate, official treatment guidelines, however influential on clinicians, are increasingly but one voice among many in a crowded arena. Sometimes, patients (and frontline clinicians) actually adopt practices like the once-a-day treatment regimen, "drug holidays" (treatment interruptions), or initiating treatment later, rather than sooner, in advance of these practices being more officially approved or advocated by researchers and guidelines (James, 2002; Lee, 2001).

Second is the rapidity with which treatment guidelines are revised–particularly around the issue of when to initiate HAART and if/when temporarily to discontinue therapy. This is understandable, given the pressures outlined above, particularly the new, experimental nature of the treatment. However, this leads to confusion, frustration, and a loss of confidence (in the value and authority of the guidelines) among patients.

One example has been the fate of the first clear treatment message of the HAART age: *hit early, hit hard.* Early euphoria over the seemingly miraculous properties of the new classes of AIDS drugs led researchers, clinicians, and clinical guidelines to call for broad, heavy use of the treatments. While some resisted the widespread enthusiasm for–and pressure to begin–the new treatment (Onstott, 1997), the majority who bowed to this pressure often suffered through complex regimens carrying severe side effects only to see medical thinking come around to the view that the treat early, treat hard approach was not supported by the evidence. Often, users grew resistant to drugs they did not yet even need to have taken (Barr, D., 2001; Goodman, 2002). This illustrates a well-established pattern in which AIDS treatments and treatment protocols have been rushed into use without solid backing of empirical evidence (Harrington, 2001; Tebas, 2001).

Among those who had already begun treatment, there has arisen a move to interrupt (temporarily or otherwise) the HAART treatment. Reasons have included: a form of respite from difficult side-effects and toxicity; improving adherence over the long term by making the regimen more bearable; and preventing or postponing development of drug resistance from excessive exposure to the drugs (Cheonis, 2000). Physicians, particularly early in this trend, generally warned against this practice (called "structured treatment interruptions" [STI] or "drug holidays"), fearing that it would reduce treatment effectiveness and breed drug resistance. However, the absence of solid scientific evidence backing their fears (while some such evidence subsequently emerged [e.g., Lawrence, Mayers, Hullsiek et al., 2003], debate persisted [Clifton, 2003; Josefson, 2003]), combined with the growing acknowledgment that many who began treatment early ended up with little to show for it save having prematurely developed drug resistance, meant their warnings often went unheeded. As one veteran treatment activist put it, "[f]ollowing the orders of the experts is largely what got us into this mess, so an anti-authority backlash should surprise no one" (Barr, M., 2001). Indeed, one AIDS doctor complained:

> My patients. . . . trust me. . . . Now, after drumming into them for four years how important it is to not miss a dose of therapy, I'm supposed to tell them, "Well, it turns out you never really needed to be on treatment in the first place?" (quoted in Barr, M., 2001)

Undermining the credibility of scientific and medical expertise is not the only result. The rapid changes in treatment guidelines, combined with the confusing mix of treatment combinations being developed to boost efficacy (while managing side-effects), can lead to uncertainty, frustration, and depression. These constitute their own form of treatment side-effects (Carter, 2002; Monroe, 2001).

The above discussion suggests at least two important implications. First, the concept of "guidelines" as we know it must be redefined, for the AIDS treatment experience is rapidly overturning some fundamental aspects of traditional guidelines. AIDS treatment protocols can no longer be seen as setting firm practice standards for years to come. Indeed, one senior figure involved in guidelines revision called the result, "a really organic document. . . . much an evolving process" (Volberding, 1999). Another put it this way: "We didn't intend it to be a cookbook. We felt that it really was an organic, viable and living document that as data came in, needed to be updated" (Goosby, 1999). In many ways, this new view of guidelines as a work in progress is realistic, even enlightened. But it remains incomplete, for it continues to regard guidelines as the sole source of treatment standards. This leads to another key shift from the traditional form of treatment guidelines: With

AIDS, official protocols may not necessarily be accepted as the ultimate authoritative source of treatment wisdom. The level of activity in the patient/activist community sometimes results in a "buzz" forming around certain drugs, drug combinations, or other aspects of treatment regimens. Such grassroots "fashions" can influence patients, thus driving physician prescribing practices. Indeed, to an extent HAART guidelines revisions, themselves, are actually being dictated, from the "bottom-up," by reports from the field of patient experiences, since the long-term, large-scale clinical trials relied upon for diseases such as cancer often simply do not exist for AIDS treatment. Finally, the basic view of protocols as establishing one central standard may be eroding, as greater attention is paid to the wide variety of patient experiences. These include issues such as side-effects, financial and other resources (some drugs require refrigeration, but some patients lack refrigerators), the local context of services and entitlements, demands of daily life, and other "idiosyncratic" factors. Perhaps it is not appropriate to set one specific treatment regimen as the standard of care for a very large category of AIDS patients.

Second, these transformations in the nature of clinical treatment guidelines lead us fundamentally to rethink the concept of adherence. After all, to *what*, exactly, are we asking patients rigidly to adhere? We strive for strict, total fulfillment of a treatment protocol, hammering home the need for 95% adherence. But this is extremely difficult to achieve in practice when, quite apart from the other burdens of treatment, the content of the treatment message evolves very rapidly, sometimes nearly completely reversing the prior message.

Nor is this limited strictly to treatment guidelines. It applies as well to HIV/AIDS prevention messages. As one experienced AIDS clinician lamented,

> We gave the mixed messages that we don't know about oral sex, we are not sure, and we've totally confused everyone. As a result, our incidence is high. I think people get frustrated and say, "Nothing is going to protect me, I might as well just do what I'm going to do." (quoted in James, 2002)

But this is merely a much-accelerated form of a more general challenge. Some public health messages are relatively simple and stable (if not always easy to carry out): quit smoking; lose weight; don't drink and drive. Messages such as these can hold fast across generations. Yet others shift substantially over time, causing frustration among the public and gradually undermining the authority of public health messages. A classic example is experts' frequently-shifting, conflicting dietary advice (Reno, 1994). With AIDS treatment, the stakes are more immediate and direct–and recommendations may shift within one year, rather than the generation or two it took nutrition messages to evolve from "eat protein" to "cut cholesterol, eat carbohydrates," to "cut carbohydrates (maybe)."

Rather than demanding utterly rigid adherence from our clients and patients, therefore, it seems more appropriate to call for *flexible rigidity*. This term reflects the changes outlined above, recognizing that the overall treatment message may need to be applied differently by different patients, to allow for individual variation in tolerating side-effects and the other demands of the regimen. It also reflects the fact that, given the confusion and uncertainty still surrounding AIDS treatment, the overall message (assuming one has in fact crystallized) may soon change. Patients and their providers must therefore be prepared to apply their rigidity somewhat selectively (i.e., customized to the specific needs of the individual patient, rather than merely automatically applying the treatment in one-size-fits-all fashion), and they must remain flexible enough to adjust rapidly to new recommendations. If, as noted above, AIDS treatment guidelines are now viewed by their architects as works in progress, so too must adherence strategies.

SUPPORTING TREATMENT CONCORDANCE IN THE HAART ERA

Taking all of these factors into consideration, the concept of concordance seems to foster the type of direct communication and negotiation needed to define and manage realistic treatment regimes. Customized treatment requires collaboration between doctor and patient to reconcile the former's pharmacologic, physiologic, and epidemiologic perspectives with the latter's lived experience of treatment, and readiness, ability, and willingness to tolerate that treatment. Moreover, since patients are generally expected to continue AIDS treatment indefinitely, and since that treatment is so prone to revision, provider-patient collaboration must be sustained throughout the treatment.

But concordance does not happen by itself, particularly where patients may be unaccustomed to conducting negotiations with their providers (Bissell, May, Noyce, 2004). If concordance is an appropriate framework through which to manage treatment decision-making, the question thus becomes: What type of organizational infrastructure is appropriate for supporting and executing a concordance approach?

Grounded as it is in the recognition of the specific (local) knowledge and expertise of patients, and complementarity between patients' and providers' expertises, treatment concordance seems an application perfectly suited to the model of inter-organization linkages–and webs of linkages–we outlined in earlier work (Rier and Indyk, this volume; Indyk and Rier, this volume[a],[b]). That work documented why and how such a model–which we have applied to improve AIDS and other sociomedical services in the inner city–taps the specific insights and other resources of community providers, academic researchers, and patients/clients, and, by constructing diverse linkages throughout the system, enables the circulation of this knowledge to, and exchange among, widely disparate sites and actors.

In fact, one particular aspect of this work is ideally designed to cultivate and maintain the sort of patient-provider relationship envisioned by the concordance approach. Space limitations preclude a proper presentation of this program, but some basics will suffice for the present discussion. The HIV Adherence Network Development (HAND) Institute is a collaboration between medical care providers, community service providers, and persons living with HIV (PLWHs). The lead agency is Mount Sinai's Designated AIDS Center, which is linked with several neighborhood health centers and community-based substance abuse programs. The HAND Institute is also linked to two HIV Care Networks, as well as to pharmacies. The target population is all PLWH served by these constituent organizations.

A recent WHO (2003:XIV) report recognized treatment adherence as a dynamic process requiring constant work. Absent a single approach or package suitable in all cases, methods must be tailored to the needs of individual patients. In particular, the report called for a fit between treatment plan and patient's stage of readiness. This is a key feature of our linkage program (Indyk and Rier, this volume [a],[b]; Indyk Coury-Doniger, Grosz et al., 1997), and is especially crucial to HAND, as demonstrated below. Much of this program's innovativeness rests on its definition of adherence not only in terms of medication dosing, scheduling, or administration, but as a *continuum* of behavior that facilitates the management of HIV disease.

The adherence literature recognizes that not all infected individuals are at a point where support with their medication regimens is even relevant. Borrowing from physical and occupational therapy, assessment tools have been developed to classify clients according to their "adherence function level" (negative, passive, co-operative, active, or proactive). Similarly, discrete elements of the treatment process have been categorized according to their "level of adherence difficulty"–i.e., the demands they place upon clients. These tasks range from those that can be met even by individuals at a "passive" functional adherence level to those requiring, for example, substantial behavior changes (such as smoking cessation) that are realistic goals only for those already at a "proactive" adherence function level (Boyer and Indyk, this volume).

Treatment adherence promotion typically focuses only on clients at one end of the continuum, those already taking combination therapy. However, HAND extends the concept of adherence support by including member agencies reaching clients at *every* stage along this adherence continuum. This extended model of treatment support is based on Prochaska and DiClemente's (1986) "stages of change" theory, which states that, for any new behavior, individuals may be located along a continuum which reflects their readiness to adopt and sustain this behavior. Prochaska and DiClemente argue that persons at different stages along the continuum require different interventions and supports to move forward. Many HIV+ individuals among the population of substance users and the homeless are not even receiving regular medical care, let alone HAART. For these individuals, the first step toward adherence is *engagement* in the medical system. The next step might be acceptance of prophylactic medications, then the acceptance of combination therapy, and so on.

HAND promotes treatment adherence by facilitating the progressive integration of adherence supports into the standard of care provided by each of its member agencies. Its Strategies Initiative identifies the unique strengths, resources, and opportunities presented by each member agency setting, and creates an action plan matching the stage (or stages) along the continuum of adherence at which the agency reaches clients. This approach is also based on a harm reduction model featuring client-centered and client-specific services reaching clients "where they are," as opposed to imposing a definition of adherence that many clients will be unable to meet. Finally, HAND's education and technical assistance arm has been named the *Learning* Center rather than *Training* Center, reflecting the philosophy that generating new knowledge, skills, and strategies for adherence requires a partnership in which clients and providers both teach and learn together.

HAND rests on the core assumption that realistic, customized regimens are impossible to achieve without sustained input from clients and patients, who must be involved in their formulation. Another core assumption, noted above, is that adherence is a continuum (ranging from engagement in regular medical care to precision in medication timing and dosage); clients thus require access to adherence support services at every point along this continuum. To put such a system into practice, HAND, like the overall linkage model more generally (Indyk and Rier, this volume [a],[b]) builds infrastructure which provides training, skill-building, technical assistance, and referral networks, and other resources to support clients, providers, and settings. An important feature of this infrastructure are forums in which providers and clients can share experiences, compare strategies, and learn from one another.

CONCLUSION

We have seen that how we think about adherence has changed significantly over time. Today, it is more widely accepted that patients have minds of their own regarding their treatment–and that, rather than automatically denying, condemning, or resisting this fact, providers can build upon it, working together with patients to negotiate a realistic, custom-tailored treatment regimen. Such a strategy, best captured by the concept of concordance, is particularly important for AIDS, where the treatments are extremely demanding, but potentially lifesaving.

At the same time, a patient-centered, custom-tailored approach must recognize that patients can be overwhelmed by their responsibility for choosing among multiple treatment options, and prefer to "[let] someone else drive" (Murray, 2003; Learned, 2003). Learned (2003), an AIDS educator, noted that not all patients actually want or can handle the empowerment of active collaboration in treatment decisions. While "knowledge is power" may indeed be the rallying cry for increasing numbers of patients nowadays, for others, "ignorance is bliss" is a better description of their preferred coping strategy. And, Learned observed, those in the two camps do not necessarily have markedly different rates of treatment success.

As discussed above, the exceptional speed with which AIDS treatment guidelines are revised (or even reversed), the controversy surrounding them, and the great variability in how patients tolerate a given treatment regimen, suggest the need to rethink the traditional goal of rigid adherence to a fixed treatment regimen. Instead, we have proposed the concept of "flexible rigidity." This highlights the need to apply individuals' adherence rigidity selectively (in custom-tailored fashion), and to remain prepared to apply it to newly-changed treatment regimens, as emerging evidence indicates.

While our discussion has focused on AIDS treatment adherence, it is relevant as well to numerous other forms of chronic diseases. The doctor-patient relationship has evolved considerably over the past two generations, and technologies such as the Internet have helped bring medical information directly into the homes of laymen (Hardey, 1999). Patients increasingly seek an active role in their treatment, and such participation could improve the selection of, and adherence to, treatment regimens. Moreover, many chronic diseases such as diabetes, hypertension, and heart disease often demand far more from patients than merely swallowing pills at appropriate intervals. Often, these involve changes in personal behaviors such as diet, exercise, and stress reduction (practices also vital, of course, to disease prevention).

With AIDS, we have learned that communicating with patients/clients, carefully assessing both their preparedness and the treatment difficulty, and then tailoring treatment to what they are ready, willing, and able to do, is a powerful strategy for helping them develop and stick to an appropriate regimen. The very same tools can be applied to helping patients stick to an appropriate diet, or reducing their smoking, or formulating a manageable hypertension medication regimen. In so doing, prevention, treatment, and services can each be made more realistic and effective.

REFERENCES

Angell, M., and Kassirer, J.P., 1994. Clinical research–What should the public believe? [editorial]. *New England Journal of Medicine 331*, 189-90.

Barr, D., 2000. Put up your nukes! *Poz.* May.

_____, 2001. Shreds of evidence. Shudda, cudda, wudda: Reevaluating the treatment revolution after the fall. *TAGline* [from the Treatment Action Group (TAG)] *8(7)* September. URL: *http://www.thebody.com/tag/sept01/evidence.html* [accessed 17 July, 2005]

Barr, M., 2001. Gimme a break! *Poz.* August. Available from URL: *http://www.poz.com/articles/_1216.shtml* [accessed 17 July, 2005]

Becker, M.H., Maiman, L.A., Kirscht, J.P., Haefner, D.P., Drachman, R.H., and Taylor, D.W., 1979. Patient compliance: Recent studies of the health belief model. p. 78-107 in R.B. Haynes, D.W. Taylor, and D.L. Sackett (Eds.), *Compliance in Health Care*. Baltimore: Johns Hopkins University Press.

Bissel, P., May, C.R., and Noyce, P.R., 2004. From compliance to concordance: Barriers to accomplishing a re-framed model of health care interactions. *Social Science & Medicine 58*, 851-62.

Boyer, A., and Indyk, D., in preparation. Poor urban women with HIV: How well is the medical community meeting their needs?

Britten, N., 2001. Prescribing and the defence of clinical autonomy. *Sociology of Health and Illness 23*, 478-96.

Carter, M., 2002. Life on HAART. *GMHC Treatment Issues 16(3)*, March. Available from URL: *http://www.thebody.com/gmhc/issues/mar02/life_on_haart.html* [accessed 17 July, 2005]

Carter, S., Taylor, D., Levenson, R., 2003. *A Question of Choice: Compliance in Medicine-taking* [second ed.; October]. Medicine Partnership. Available from: URL *http://easi.negrisud.it/etica/DWL/CP/OI/aquestionofchoice.pdf [accessed 17 July, 2005]*

Cheonis, N., 2000. Structured treatment interruption: Future protocol or wishful thinking? *Bulletin of Experimental Treatments for AIDS* [San Francisco AIDS Foundation]. Spring. Available from: URL *http://www.sfaf.org/treatment/beta/b43/b43 interrupt.html [accessed* 17 July, 2005]

Chesney, M.A., 2003. Adherence to HAART Regimens. *AIDS Patient Care and STDs 17*, 169-77.

Chesney, M.A., Morin, M., Sherr, L., 2000. Adherence to HIV therapy combination treatment. *Social Science & Medicine 50*, 1599-1605.

Clifton, C.E., 2003. To break or not to break, that is still the question. *Positively Aware* [Test Positive Aware Network] Sept./Oct. Available from URL *http://www.thebody. com/tpan/septoct_03/interruption.html* [accessed 17 July, 2005]

Conrad, P., 1985. The meaning of medication: Another look at compliance. *Social Science & Medicine 20*, 29-37.

Donovan, J.L., and Blake, D.R., 1992. Patient non-compliance: Deviance or reasoned decision-making? *Social Science & Medicine 34*, 507-13.

Gilden, D., 1998. The latest on early intervention. *Poz* (October).

Goodman, L., 2002. The problem with protease. *Poz*. September. Available from URL: *http://www.poz.com/articles/_944.shtml* [accessed 17 July, 2005].

Goosby, E., 1999. *Revisions and Anticipated Changes to the Federal Guidelines for the Treatment of HIV*. Comments delivered on HIV Treatment Live! Internet tele-conference sponsored by HIVandHepatitis.com, hosted by Ron Baker, May 10.

Hardey, M., 1999. Doctor in the house: The Internet as a source of lay health knowledge and the challenge to expertise. *Sociology of Health and Illness 21*, 820-35.

Harrington, M., 2001. Hit Hard, Later . . . ? *GMHC [Gay Men's Health Crisis] Treatment Issues. 15(2/3[Feb./March])*. Available from URL: *http://www.thebody. com/gmhc/issues/feb_mar01/hit.html* [accessed 17 July, 2005]

Hulka, B.S., 1979. Patient-clinician interactions and compliance. pp. 63-77 in R.B. Haynes, D.W. Taylor, and D.L. Sackett (Eds.), *Compliance in Health Care*. Baltimore: Johns Hopkins University Press.

Indyk, D., Coury-Doniger, P., Grosz, J., Pruden, S., Jordan, S., Kaudeyr, K., Edwards, T., Klein, S., Stevens, P.C., 1997. HIV prevention: Applying "stages of change" theory to accelerate bottom-up and top-down prevention knowledge production and technology transfer. Presented at the Public Health Conference on Records and Statistics and the National Committee on Vital and Health Statistics. Washington, D.C., July.

Indyk, D., and Rier, D.A., 1993. Grassroots AIDS knowledge: Implications for the boundaries of science and collective action. *Knowledge: Creation, Diffusion, Utilization 15*, 3-43.

Indyk, D., and Rier, D.A., 2005. Wiring the HIV/AIDS system: Building interorganizational infrastructure to link people, sites, and networks. *Social Work in Health Care 42* (3/4), 29-45.

Indyk, D., and Rier, D.A., 2005. Requisites, benefits, and challenges of sustainable HIV/AIDS system-building: Where theory meets practice. *Social Work in Health Care 42* (3/4), 93-110.

James, J.S., 2002. HIV medicine after Barcelona conference: Interview with Howard Grossman, M.D. *AIDS Treatment News #383 (6 September)*. Available from URL: *http://www.thebody.com/atn/383/interview.html* [accessed 17 July, 2005]

Josefson, D., 2003. Breaks from antiretroviral treatment are not the answer for HIV patients. *British Medical Journal 327(6 September)*, 520.

Karwal, A.K., Verkaik, R., and Jansen, C., 2000. Non-adherence to procedures: Why does it happen? pp. 139-56 in *Safety: Beginning at the Top*. Proceedings of the 12th Annual European Aviation Seminar. March 6-8, Amsterdam.

Lawrence, J., Mayers, D.L., Hullsiek, K.H., Collins, G., Abrams, D.I., Reisler, R.B, Crane, L.R., Schmetter, B.S., Dionne, T.J., Saldanha, J.M., Jones, M.C., Baxter, J.D., 2003. Structured treatment interruption in patients with multidrug-resistant Human Immunodeficiency Virus. *New England Journal of Medicine 349(August 28)*, 837-46.

Learned, J., 2003. Starting, switching, stopping: Personal perspectives on making treatment decisions. *ACRIA [AIDS Community Research Initiative of America] Update 12 (3 [Summer])*. Available from URL *http://www.thebody.com/cria/ summer03/learned. html.* [accessed 17 July, 2005]

Lee, D. 2001. Change of HAART. *Poz*. May. Available from URL: *http://www.poz. com/articles/_1170.shtml* [accessed 17 July, 2005]

Lerner, B.H., Gulick, R.M., and Dubler, N.N., 1998. Rethinking nonadherence: Historical perspectives on triple-drug therapy for HIV disease. *Annals of Internal Medicine 129(7)*, 573-78.

Milano, M., 2001. Living with guidelines: A personal perspective. *CRIA [AIDS Community Research Initiative of America] Update 10(2)[Spring]*. URL: *http://www.thebody. com/cria/spring01/guidelines.html* [accessed 17 July, 2005]

Monroe, A., 2001. Psychological issues and HIV: Dealing with the uncertainty of changing treatment strategies [Community Forum Summary]. *AIDS Community Research Initiative of America*. March. Available from URL: *http://www.thebody.com/cria/forums/psychology.html* [accessed 17 July, 2005]

Murray, C., 2003. Letting someone else drive. *ACRIA [AIDS Community Research Initiative of America] Update 12(3) Summer*. Available from URL: *http://www.thebody.com/ cria/summer03/murray.html* [accessed 17 July, 2005]

Onstott, M., 1997. The defiant ones. *Poz*. October.

Palella, F.J., Jr, Delaney, K.M., Moorman, A.C., Loveless, M.O., Fuhrer, J., Satten, G.A. et al., 1998. Declining morbidity and mortality among patients with advanced human immunodeficiency virus infection. HIV outpatient study investigators. *New England Journal of Medicine 338*, 853-60.

Prochaska, J.O., & DiClemente, C.C., 1986. Toward a comprehensive model of change. pp. 3-27 in W.R. Miller and N. Heather (Eds.), *Treating addictive behaviors: Processes of change*. NY: Plenum Press.

Remien, R.H., Hirky, A.E., Johnson, M.O., Weinhardt, L.S., Whittier, D., and Le, G.M. 2003. Adherence to medication treatment: A qualitative study of facilitators and barriers among a diverse sample of HIV+ men and women in four U.S. cities. *AIDS and Behavior 7*, 61-72.

Reno, R., 1994. Spare us the bad news on food—We don't care. *New York Newsday* August 25, p. A49.

Rier, D.A., and Indyk, D., this volume. The rationale of interorganizational linkages to connect multiple sites of expertise, knowledge production, and knowledge transfer: An example from HIV/AIDS services for the inner city. Accepted for publication in *Social Work in Health Care*.

Sackett, D.L., Snow, J.C., 1979. The magnitude of compliance and noncompliance. pp. 11-22 in R.B. Haynes, D.W. Taylor, and D.L. Sackett (Eds.), *Compliance in Health Care*. Baltimore: Johns Hopkins University Press.

Steiner, J.F., and Earnest, M.A., 2000. The language of medication-taking. *Annals of Internal Medicine 132(11)*, 926-30.

Svarstad, B.L., 1976. Physician-patient communication and patient conformity with medical advice. pp. 220-38 in D. Mechanic (Ed.), *The Growth of Bureaucratic Medicine*. NY: John Wiley & Sons.

Tebas, P., 2001. The 1st International AIDS Society Conference on HIV Pathogenesis and Treatment: IAS-USA panel. 10 July. *The Body*. Available from URL: *http://www.thebody.com/confs/ias2001/tebas7.html* [accessed 17 July, 2005]

Townsend, A., Hunt, K., and Wyke, S., 2003. Managing multiple morbidity in mid-life: A qualitative study of attitudes to drug use. *British Medical Journal 327*, 837-40.

Van Servellen, G., Chang, B., Garcia, L., and Lombardi, E., 2002. Individual and system level factors associated with treatment nonadherence in Human Immunodeficiency Virus-infected men and women. *AIDS Patient Care and STDs 16*, 269-81.

Volberding, P.A., 1999. Revisions and anticipated changes to the federal guidelines for the treatment of HIV. Comments delivered on HIV Treatment Live! Internet tele-conference sponsored by HIVandHepatitis.com, hosted by Ron Baker, May 10.

WHO, 2003. *Adherence to long-term therapies: Evidence for action*. Available from URL: *http://www.who.int/chronic_conditions/en/adherence_report.pdf* [accessed 17 July, 2005]

Weiss, M., Britten, N., 2003. What is concordance? *The Pharmaceutical Journal 271*, 493.

Working Party, 1997. From compliance to concordance: Achieving shared goals in medicine taking. Report of the Working Party. London: Royal Pharmaceutical Society of Great Britain/Merck, Sharpe, and Dohme. Available from URL: *http://www.medicines-partnership.org/about-us/history-context* [accessed 17 July, 2005]

Zola, I.K., [1981]1987. Structural constraints in the doctor-patient relationship: The case of non-compliance. pps. 203-09 in H.D. Schwartz (Ed.), *Dominant Issues in Medical Sociology* [2nd ed.]. NY: Random House.

Shaping Garments of Care:
Tools for Maximizing Adherence Potential

Ann Boyer, MD
Debbie Indyk, PhD

SUMMARY. There is a tendency in health care to treat clients' maladies in accordance with two basic premises: (1) the medical needs of the client (as perceived by the clinician) can be successfully addressed by focusing solely on that aspect of the client's life and (2) if the client is not able or ready, then there will be someone in the client's support system to take responsibility for administering prescribed therapy. In many cases these assumptions hold true, but for certain sub-populations they do not, notably: individuals with substandard/chaotic lives, those with multiple confounding diagnoses (mental health, substance abuse, disability, addiction, domestic violence) who have neither personal adherence ability nor adequate support systems. They are rarely seen in ambulatory care settings, engaging with the health care system only through emergency rooms and hospital admissions. Such a group makes up a large proportion of urban, HIV positive clients. For them, successful adherence can only be accomplished by rethinking what constitutes 'care' and 'tailoring' that care to the individual. In this context adherence requires the interweaving of three sets of needs: (1) needs perceived by the client, (2) client needs as observed by an objective recorder and

---

Ann Boyer, MD, and Debbie Indyk, PhD, are affiliated with the Mount Sinai School of Medicine, New York, NY.

[Haworth co-indexing entry note]: "Shaping Garments of Care: Tools for Maximizing Adherence Potential." Boyer, Ann, and Debbie Indyk. Co-published simultaneously in *Social Work in Health Care* (The Haworth Press, Inc.) Vol. 42, No. 3/4, 2006, pp. 151-166; and: *The Geometry of Care: Linking Resources, Research, and Community to Reduce Degrees of Separation Between HIV Treatment and Prevention* (ed: Debbie Indyk) The Haworth Social Work Practice Press, an imprint of The Haworth Press, Inc., 2006, pp. 151-166. Single or multiple copies of this article are available for a fee from The Haworth Document Delivery Service [1-800-HAWORTH, 9:00 a.m. - 5:00 p.m. (EST). E-mail address: docdelivery@haworthpress.com].

doi:10.1300/J010v42n03_10

assessed for impact on the client's ability and willingness to be adherent and (3) medical needs identified by a clinician. Extensive work with this population has led to the creation of a Cluster of Tools (HIVCOT), designed to quantitatively assess the severity of the varied needs (Health Importance Level or HIL), the adherence ability of the client (Adherence Functional Level or AFL) and how difficult it is to adhere to a given treatment (Level of Adherence Difficulty or LAD). Through the application of these tools it becomes possible for the medical providers to make individual adjustments to the design of care so that it closely fits the needs and abilities of the client. In this way the likelihood of adherence is maximized. *[Article copies available for a fee from The Haworth Document Delivery Service: 1-800-HAWORTH. E-mail address: <docdelivery@haworth press.com> Website: <http://www.HaworthPress.com> © 2006 by The Haworth Press, Inc. All rights reserved.]*

KEYWORDS. Adherence, functional scales, co-morbidities, client-centered

The introduction of HAART has placed HIV in the category of controllable chronic illnesses. As such, the greatest single factor determining long-term outcomes is adherence to treatment (Paterson, Swindells, Mohr et al., 2000; Chesney, Morin, and Sherr, 2000). In recent years adherence has become easier for most chronic diseases through simplified regimens (less pills, less frequent dosing) and decreased unpleasant side effects. However, HIV differs from other chronic illnesses in two areas that strongly effect adherence success. The first is *degree of adherence.* In most chronic illnesses, continued improvement in adherence parallels improvement in the condition. In HIV treatment there is no opportunity to gradually improve your adherence. Poor adherence is associated with virologic and immunologic failure and clinical disease progression as well as development of drug resistance (Sethi, 2004).

The second is the *population profile* (Delor & Hubert, 2000; Broadhead, Heckathorn, & Altice, 2002; Bouhnik, Chesney, Carrieri et al., 2002). A high percentage of HIV infected persons have a history of disadvantaged/chaotic, trauma-filled lives with multiple confounding diagnoses (serious mental health, substance use, psychosocial, cognitive or geriatric issues, disabilities, addictions), many lack adequate food, clothing and housing, and most lack adequate social support systems.

Each of these unmet or unmeetable needs reduces the probability of successful, consistent care and treatment–reduces 'the functional level' of the person in terms of adherence. As a result, these clients are rarely seen in ambulatory care settings because chronic medical issues are low on their personal list of needs, or because their level of function is inadequate for them to make and keep regular appointments. They engage with the health care system through emergency rooms and hospital admissions only when incapacitated or intolerably symptomatic. When they are symptomatically improved, they return to their previous life-style.

In this population, then, successful adherence encompasses much more than the traditional concept of compliance to standardized treatment recommendations or provider guidelines (Ickovics & Meade, 2002; Ammassari, Trotta, Murri et al., 2002). A positive, long-term impact on their health can only occur if other overshadowing needs in their lives are first taken into account, and then a medical care plan is tailored to the level at which they are currently functioning. Such an approach is not without precedent: in the fields of Physical and Occupational Medicine: The functional level of the patient is evaluated *before* prescribing therapy, and the level of difficulty of the therapy is tailored to that individual's functional level. Modification of therapy over time is determined by measurable changes in client physical and neurological function.

A difficulty in applying this model to other areas of medicine has been the lack of objective measures of functional status (as it relates to potential adherence). One common denominator affecting people's motivation and ability to function across different medical and cultural areas is 'burden of need.' The more basic, immediate and complex his needs, the more difficulty the person is likely to have with adherence. An estimate of the weight of the burden of need at a given time can be used to predict the degree of assistance a person will require in order to achieve successful adherence.

Through work with marginalized, HIV-positive individuals living in New York City, the authors have developed and implemented an HIV Cluster of Tools (HIVCOT) designed to match the level of difficulty involved in adhering to treatment with a person's functional level (in terms of degree of assistance a person is likely to require in order to be adherent). The tools are needs-based, with needs assessments being incorporated from different perspectives. Successful adherence to medical care and

treatment involves weaving together three sets of interdependent needs:
(a) needs perceived by the client, (b) client needs observed by an objective recorder (and assessed for impact on the client's ability to be adherent) and (c) medical needs identified by a clinician. The first two sets of needs are stratified according to Maslow's needs hierarchy (Heylighen, 1992) and are rated in terms of their potential impact on adherence to medical therapy (Adherence Functional Level or AFL) The composite score (0-4) reflects the degree of support that person will require for successful adherence, and ranges from 1, 'Passive' (requiring complete physical support–as in a skilled nursing facility) to 4, 'Pro-active' (totally independent). The third needs assessment–medical needs–are examined to determine (a) how critical each medical need is (Health Importance Level or HIL) and (b) how difficult it will be to adhere to treatment for that need (Level of Adherence Difficulty or LAD). The LAD uses the same scoring scale as the AFL, estimating what level of independence is required to be adherent to that treatment plan as it is normally administered. It then becomes possible to see if there is a discrepancy between AFL and LAD, and assess the feasibility of making adjustments in the therapy to reduce the LAD to accommodate a lower functional level (introducing DOT, for example, which drops the LAD by assisting the client with taking medication on a daily basis).

At the core of HIVCOT are two concepts. First, adherence is dynamically balanced between the level of adherence difficulty (how hard it is to adhere to the total treatment 'package') and the client's adherence functional level (how motivated and capable he is). Second, the level of adherence achieved at any given time depends on the clinician's accurate tailoring of total planned treatment to the client's current capability.

This paper advances the proposition that such an approach in other areas of medicine may lead to improved client adherence and, consequently, health and care. This approach becomes even more vital given the extent to which the locus of control over HIV treatment and prevention continues to shift toward the HIV-positive individuals themselves (Indyk & Golub, this volume). Such a shift in locus requires a shift in approach to supporting HIV adherence and understanding adherence in the context of a patient's complete life.

THE TOOLS

The first step in the HIVCOT process is to document the client's current needs from three vantage points and integrate this information into HIVCOT: (a) Client *perceived*–these needs are listed in the client's words and prioritized by the client; (b) *observed* needs assessed by an objective recorder during a client interview (if possible, in the client's environs); and (c) medically *determined* need based on objective data–history, physical examination, and laboratory studies.

Both perceived and observed needs are stratified according to Maslow's needs hierarchy: (1) physiological needs; (2) safety needs; (3) needs for love, affection and sense of belonging; (4) needs for esteem and (5) needs for self-actualization (Heylighen, 1992) and are rated in terms of their potential impact on adherence to medical therapy (see Table 1).

The second step in HIVCOT is to use the rated perceived and observed needs as part of the assessment of the patient's Adherence Functional Level (AFL). AFL is a numerical estimate of the level at which one would expect a client to function with respect to managing medical treatment.

The third step in HIVCOT is to prioritize the medically observed needs according to degree of life-impact each condition is expected to have. This constitutes the Health Importance Level (HIL). Often a client has so many medical needs that to be adherent to all treatment requires an unattainable functional level. For this reason it is important to be able to prioritize by Health Importance Level and begin by addressing those of highest importance (see Table 2 which offers scale-based rating to be assigned by a clinician).

The final step in HIVCOT is to select out all the HIL 3-4 medical needs and examine the complexity and difficulty of the standard treatment for them–separately and together. This is the expected Level of Adherence Difficulty (LAD) and is scored similarly to the Adherence Functional Level (see Table 3). If the LAD is higher than the AFL, then successful adherence is unlikely, but through creative solutions to lower LADs and attention to client needs so as to raise the AFL, good adherence can be accomplished.

Using this approach, the needs as perceived by the client and observed by the staff are identified, prioritized and categorized according to: (1) how basic the need is to the survival of the person (e.g., food is a level 1 need), and (2) how difficult will it be for the *for the individual to get the need met* (i.e., how easily attainable is it by this person at this time). Finally, a service model is created for each client–thus placing solutions to needs within a client's reach (see Table 4).

Examples of how this method has been applied are described in the case studies below:

TABLE 1. Adherence Functional Levels

Level	Definition	Observational Cues
0 - Negative	Unwilling to interact, hostile, opposes any approach by unfamiliar persons.	
1 - Passive	Essentially the status of someone in a Skilled Nursing Facility: limited consciousness or physical ability, accepts ministrations and medication as DOT if taken to the client.	a) unkempt appearance or disordered physical environment b) apparent depression c) apparent uncontrolled physical or mental disorder d) mistrust of the need for/helpfulness of medical treatment e) presence of any 'physiologic' perceived or observed needs (food, warm clothing...)
2 - Cooperative	Able to make him/herself available (i.e., to come to designated site) for interaction (including pick-ups for appointments by escorts, administration of therapy such as meds, dressing changes, etc). May be able to take medication fairly consistently (especially if reminded) and to adhere to DOT in conjunction with another program (such as MMTP).	a) apparent dementia b) unstable housing c) active substance use d) history of health neglect *May require additional assistance to reach Level 3 if...* a) intellectually challenged b) literacy limited
3 - Active	Able and willing to follow a schedule of health care, including administration of necessary medications, as long as demands are not extreme.	a) has demonstrated the willingness to participate in other chronic illness care b) demonstrates an interest in managing his/her health care
4 - Proactive	Seeks care for all medical issues. Actively involved in independent living, forward thinking which includes making and keeping appointments, able to maintain a routine of daily life.	

CASE STUDIES

Low AFL, high LAD. This a 52-year-old African-American male, HIV+ and HCV+, with a high viral load and CD4 215, who was actively using subcutaneous cocaine and heroin, resulting in the development of numerous injection-site abscesses. Always pleasant when visited at his Single-Room-Occupancy (SRO) hotel by Health Bridge personnel, he was frequently entertaining guests and was not interested in engaging in medical care, even with an escort. His AFL was therefore less than 1. Over time he agreed to reduce his substance use and, through Health Bridge, joined the methadone maintenance treatment program (MMTP)

TABLE 2. Health Importance Level

Level	Definition
HIL 1	Can improve life quality, e.g., regular exercise, psychotherapy, acupuncture, stress reduction modalities
HIL 2	May negatively impact longevity or quality of life, e.g., smoking, any alcohol use by a person with Hepatitis C, decreased folate, constipation, dental caries, overweight, elevated cholesterol.
HIV 3	Long term life-threatening, e.g., lack of prophylaxis and treatment in a client with advanced HIV, lack of regular medical care and support for chronic physical or debilitating mental illness (hypertension, diabetes, major depression...)
HIL 4	Immediately, or in the short term life-threatening, e.g.: untreated acute infection in a client with advanced HIV, severe anemia, suicidal ideation, drug overdose, need for anti-coagulation.

TABLE 3. Level of Adherence Difficulty

Level	Care that Can Be Provided	Requires at Least AFL
LAD 0	None – Client refuses all care.	0 - Negative
LAD 1	a) Acute support/rewards (e.g., food, bandages, a validating presence for disclosures of personal trauma/frustration, escort to E.R. or a detoxification program); b) Care which can be given by a single intervention that is less negative than the state before the intervention (e.g., acute medical care); c) Care requiring minimal responsible behavior by the client (supportive living, supportive medical care, on-site DOT)	1 - Passive
LAD 2	a) Care which involves willingness and ability to keep appointments when reminded and escorted (reactivating Medicaid, improving housing, primary and specialty medical care, attending a day program) or to learn/develop skills (basic life skills, reading); b) Care requiring short term behavioral change (drug detoxification/rehabilitation, a limited course of antibiotics); c) Care which can be effective at < 95% adherence levels (eg: treatment for HTN or DM, prophylaxis for Opportunistic Infections); off-site DOT (in an MMTP or other daily program)	2 - Cooperative
LAD 3	a) Care requiring integration of planning, routinizing and habit-formation skills as well as a consistent daily schedule (ART, steady employment, independent living)	3 - Active
LAD 4	a) Care requiring a behavior change in which negative or uncertain reinforcement replaces neutral or positive reinforcement (smoking cessation, treatment with unpleasant side effects such as that for Hepatitis C), b) Care requiring complex life, negotiating and planning skills and future thinking	4 - Proactive

at Mount Sinai. He continued to inject cocaine, but was not as frequently impaired, was very consistent about attending his methadone program and became more involved in keeping medical appointments and engaging in activities suggested by Health Bridge. His AFL had thus risen to above 2. Early in 2002, he presented to Mount Sinai Emergency Room gravely ill with what was found to be tubercular pericarditis. He slowly recovered and returned home on DOT for his TB medication (LAD of 2, requiring only cooperative, Level 2 function). His near-death experience affected him and he became more concerned about taking care of his health and beginning ART. Unfortunately, he had also developed progressive dementia. When there was no longer someone to remind him and give him his pills at least once a day (which was done for the first month) he forgot more and more often, and the ART was stopped because of concerns about the development of viral resistance. Independently taking daily medication for a prolonged period has an LAD of 3, requiring an 'active' AFL of 3–but the presence of significant dementia makes it extremely unlikely that this client would be capable of that level of function, at least until the dementia is reversed by appropriate ART. Early in 2004, he developed a recurrence of tuberculosis and was again begun on DOT. Recently, after having been on TB medications for 18 months, he was re-evaluated and it was the medical consensus that his immune system was so suppressed by HIV (CD4 < 100) that he could never be taken off DOT unless his HIV was controlled. Through extensive negotiations with the NYCDOH a plan was devised: each day, when he is seen in his SRO for his DOT, he is reminded to take his HIV medications (which are individual-dose packaged and need to be taken only once a day). It has therefore been possible to drop the LAD to 2–the same as his AFL–and he has not missed a dose so far. Each time we visit him, he proudly displays his pill packs to show how many he has taken.

Raising AFL through attention to competing concerns. SH is a 38-year-old Hispanic woman with multiple medical problems including advanced HIV (low CD4, high viral load), cervical carcinoma treated shortly before we met her, malodorous purulent gingivitis and recurrent severe diarrhea. Additionally she had longstanding, untreated PTSD/chronic depression and used alcohol and crack-cocaine to self-medicate the symptoms. At the time of engagement in an SRO to which she had recently moved from a Skilled Nursing Facility her AFL was 0 (refusing all care), and her most pressing *self-perceived* needs were "fixing [her] teeth." and "getting [her] kids back." Her most immediate *observed need* was for support/relief from her guilt and pain related to los-

TABLE 4. Matching Needs with Adherence Functional Levels

NEED	CAN BE MET WITH AFL 1	CAN BE MET WITH AFL 2	CAN BE MET WITH AFL 3
HIV PROPHYLAXIS	DOT on site (Home or SNF)	DOT at MMTP or other frequented venue	Self medication[1], best if given pillbox and other supports
ART	Same as above .	Same as above	Same as above
Health care and monitoring	Home visits	Appointments made for client, reminders given, escorted	Attends appointments independently–may need assistance with multiple or complex schedule
Anticoagulation	DOT on site, blood samples drawn on site weekly	DOT on site or other venue, escort weekly for blood work	Self medicates, independently comes for weekly blood work
Chronic illness (e.g., Diabetes, Hypertension)	DOT and monitoring on site	DOT on site or other venue, teach and review home monitoring, make appointments and escort for related health care	Self medicates and monitors. Attends appointments independently
Serious, urgent medical issues (e.g., evidence of malignancy)	Education and persuasion on site	Make and escort to appointments	Attends appointments independently–may need assistance with multiple or complex schedule
Emergent medical issues (e.g., prolonged diarrhea, cough and fever)	On site persuasion to accept ambulance transport	Client taken to hospital by ambulance called on site or is escorted to Urgent Care	Client comes to Urgent Care independently before an ambulance is necessary

[1]AFL 4 required if other prescriptions are given complicating regimen.

ing her children and her own childhood trauma. By arranging for immediate individual counseling for her PTSD/child loss issues and escorted treatment for her gingivitis, Health Bridge personnel succeeded in gaining, first her trust, and then her commitment to try to care for herself more. She began on helpful psychotropic medication, progressed to an AFL of 2, decreased her substance use, but was unable to take ART as prescribed. She desperately wanted to achieve that degree of independence–she had bags of medication in drawers, under her bed, in the refrigerator and would take them willingly if someone went to her room and reminded her–but due to her chaotic life-style and some intellectual limitations, she could not consistently take them on her own. The same was true for the necessary diet restrictions required for her lactose-intolerant diarrhea. She ultimately agreed to enter a care facility where she could be monitored for medication and diet but still go and come and be involved in numerous activities. She did extremely well there. Thus her AFL remained at 2, but the LAD was reduced to the same level through placement in a supportive facility.

Managing LAD in the face of disease progression. LI is a 42-year-old African American woman, HIV+, HCV+ (high viral load and CD4 < 10), with severe asthma, anemia, cachexia, multiple hospitalizations for PCP0. Her mental health issues included a long history of depression/schizophrenia/PTSD, she was a chronic user of heroin and cocaine. and was first engaged when she and her discordant partner of 11 years were admitted to the MMTP at Mount Sinai. At the time of engagement she was homeless, without food, from another state with no benefits, no medical care and probable pneumonia. Her *self-perceived needs* were for food, shelter and entitlements. Her AFL was 1. Additional high-priority *observed needs* included hospital admission for her pneumonia and a stable living arrangement on discharge. She agreed to hospital admission and was treated for PCP (LAD 1, passive). On discharge she was assisted by Health Bridge to begin medical and psychiatric care, obtained documentation for receiving HASA services, was coached through the process of establishing a legal domestic partnership (so that she and her partner would be housed together) and began receiving public assistance. Partial stabilization of her life style resulted, but the instability of her housing continued as she and her partner were shifted every 28 days–at one point to a hotel from which they returned after one day with total-body bedbug bites, and at no point to an environment in which she and her partner could cook healthy regular meals and engage in a healthy life-style or regular taking of medication. For these reasons, she was unable to move beyond an AFL of 1-2, and there was nothing in place to provide her with daily adherence reminders, which would reduce the LAD to match the AFL. She had two more admissions for PCP, was told by her primary care provider that she was 'killing herself' (which is probably true, because, with her depression, she did not care about living) and had a psychotic break because she discontinued her psychotropic medication. She was eventually placed in a SNF, where she did very well (LAD 1). She left, relapsed to drug use, and was hospitalized for severe pneumonia and intractable asthma. She stabilized medically and attention was focused on treating her mental health issues and restarting her on methadone. Her outlook improved, depression lifted, and she began to take more of an interest in her own health (AFL 2). She is currently living with supportive family members, has VNS (combined LAD 2) and continues to do well.

Achieving an AFL of 4. YV is a 34-year-old Hispanic woman who was diagnosed with both HIV and breast cancer while in rehabilitation for heroin and cocaine use 5 years ago. She underwent a radical mastectomy, chemotherapy, was counseled on HIV therapy and discharged from the facility with no follow-up for either problem. Not surprisingly, she relapsed. Following a later incarceration, during which she received ART, she again relapsed and was mandated by parole to enter a methadone program or return to jail. At the time she was admitted to the MMTP at Mount Sinai, she was hungry, homeless with no support services, suffered from major depression and had a 9-year-old daughter who had been removed and sent to live with YV's disapproving sister. Her AFL was 1–passive, and her immediate *perceived needs* (though unfocused and confused) seemed to be the basic necessities of food, clothing and shelter. Other *observed needs* included assistance in getting entitlements and services and a profound need for warm support and advocacy–her feelings of inadequacy and powerlessness were paralyzing to any forward initiatives to improve her life or health. Since then, she has received intense and unfailing support from Health Bridge and, through HB, from the Fortune Society, a primary care provider and psychiatrist in the AIDS center at Mount Sinai–HB personnel have gone out to her, wherever she was (shelter, SRO) and supported her as she gradually began to believe in herself and her capabilities. As a result, she has risen to AFL 3-4, is successfully adherent to ART on her own, makes and keeps her appointments. She now lives independently in an apartment with her daughter, is in good psychological and medical health and is doing extremely well.

LAD failure. MA was a 37-year-old, slim, active, energetic Hispanic woman HIV+, HCV+, high viral load, CD4 < 150, moderate to severe asthma, who was first engaged seeking treatment in the methadone program at Mount Sinai. Her AFL was 0, resistant to any care. Shortly after joining the program, she was seen and referred to the Emergency Room with probable pneumonia. She refused admission to Mount Sinai but received prescriptions for antibiotics from another ER (LAD 3), which she did not take. She returned 5 days later and accepted admission to Mount Sinai where she was treated for PCP (LAD 1, in hospital–passive). She was discharged on a Saturday, when it was too late to receive a bottle of methadone for Sunday. On Sunday, she used heroin and cocaine to combat withdrawal and suffered an M.I. (almost surely because of the cocaine) and was readmitted to Mount Sinai. That evening, she underwent a cardiac catheterization and stent placement. She was discharged 5 days later with a serious cardiac diagnosis (HIL 4) on coumadin and digoxin (LAD 3-4) to temporary housing with two bed-ridden relatives that she had previously cared for, and who expected her to care for them again. She was, at that point, quite cooperative (AFL 2), but did re-fuse daily VNS (which would have reduced the LAD to 2) because she was "just there temporarily and [didn't] want to cause no bother." Numerous attempts were made during this time to get her into a setting where she could be given her medication at the appro-priate times each day (LAD 1-2). She went to the requested meetings but there were delays from the facility administration. She was hos-pitalized for a second M.I. in the ICU of another hospital. When she was discharged she was given prescriptions for 10 different medica-tions, at least two of which were the life-essential: digoxin and coumadin. Again, she had no assistance in obtaining, prioritizing or taking the medications, just a large handful of prescriptions (LAD > 4). She arrived DOA at a hospital 2 days later. Here was a person with an AFL of 2, who was required to function at a level 4, or die–so she died.

Addressing child care needs as a path to raising AFL. NC is a 40-year-old HIV+ Hispanic woman who, at the time of engagement, had a CD4 of 161, moderate asthma, smoked 1 pack of cigarettes per day, and was not in medical care. Her mental health issues included depression, anxiety, PTSD from untreated childhood sexual abuse and agoraphobia. She was in fragile recovery from alcohol and crack-cocaine use. She was first engaged when she came to a community-based organization request-ing nursing and social work assistance for her 3 young-adult children with severe developmental or emotional problems her highest priority *perceived need* was for care assistance with her three disabled children. The most immediate *observed need* was support and stabilization of her mental health issues which, in addition to the above, included concerns that she had only completed 6th grade and felt acutely uncomfortable about her literacy level (no HIL above 2) and, because of her many other issues, her Functional Adherence Level was low, (between 1 and 2–pas-sive to cooperative) because of her inability to leave home or deal with regimens at home without support. By pursuing her highest priority *perceived need* of child care, trust was gained, and after almost a year, she gave permis-sion to bring psychiatric care to her home and she began therapy. Later, she be-gan medication and is now able to leave home and travel on public transportation. She is in consistent HIV care on ART and is actively supported to become involved in a mothers' group at a CBO.

DISCUSSION

Successful treatment of HIV demands near-perfect adherence to a repetitive routine of scheduled behavior from a population made up largely of persons with chaotic life styles and more immediate, pressing priorities than their long term health adherence (Paterson, Swindells, Mohr et al., 2000; Bouhnik, Chesney, Carrieri et al., 2002). Providers can overcome this disparity by weaving together the medically-determined 'urgent needs' and the client-determined 'urgent needs': attending first to client-perceived urgent needs, reducing the most needed adherence behavior to a form within the capability of the client and making it part of a complete 'garment of care,' tailored to the individual.

Discussion with, and observation of a client, can yield a clear picture of what the client sees as important components of that garment, and what additional care 'pieces' the observer feels are indicated. With perceived and observed needs in mind, it is possible to estimate the Adherence Functional Level of that person at that point in time.

Review by a medical provider of the client's comprehensive health data will enable him to list all diagnoses and assign each a Health Importance Level. Once the client's health status has been assessed, treatment regimens for all diagnoses with HIL 3-4 should be examined for Level of Adherence Difficulty. If the LAD is any degree higher than the client's current AFL, adherence is highly unlikely. High urgency for medical treatment, as indicated by a level 4, would normally be addressed first. By eliminating obstacles (e.g.: arranging for home delivery of medication) and reducing to a minimum other medication (addressing HIL 1 or 2 issues such as vitamin or mineral deficiency later) the LAD may be lowered to be within the range of the client's AFL. But, if it is not, then every attempt should be made to reduce the LAD to within the client's capacity by other means. One way to accomplish this is to send the client to a Skilled Nursing Facility (SNF). A problem with this type of disposition is that the client with advanced HIV may do well under 'passive' care–but he is not developing coping skills and may well return to his unsupported, chaotic life and baseline AFL if he leaves. There are also a number of clients who reject the idea of a SNF. There are other ways to reduce LAD: besides delivery and reducing number of pills and frequency to a minimum: package all pills for each dose together, DOT on site, DOT at a methadone, day program or clinic, daily reminders to clients at home to take their meds. (Ickovics & Meade, 2002a; Tuldra & Wu, 2002)

When a client has *no* HIL above 3, he has a 'health margin'–there is time to work with other aspects of his 'garment of care' to increase his AFL before it becomes a vital issue. And, as he approaches an AFL of 3 (that necessary to adhere to simplified ART) efforts can be put into simplifying and 'fitting' the regimen to him. Table 4 provides examples of how the HIL need can be met to support various adherence functional levels.

Bridging the Adherence Gap

One key concept related to this approach is that people do not manage HIV infection any differently than they manage the rest of their lives. Today, the growing number of individuals with HIV challenges society as to how to (1) reduce disease progression, (2) promote health maintenance and (3) support behaviors which reduce the risk of acquisition and transmission of additional infection–in a population for whom HIV occupies a close-to-last position on its priority list. The goal of treating HIV still exists, but it must go far beyond prescribing anti-retroviral therapy, information about and encouragement to practice harm-reducing behaviors and good health measures. It must engage the clients "where they're at" (geographically, emotionally, priority-wise) and strive to partner them into becoming active participants in their own care. This can only occur if their priorities are addressed, issues validated, basic life needs met and functional limitations taken into account. To do this one must assess needs, readiness, skills and resources of clients, both medical and emotional, and tailor any care plan to the complex multiple factors that make up the individual's life and person.

Management of HIV can be prescribed by medical providers, but it must be accomplished through client "adherence" to these recommendations. Individuals need to be supported in their acceptance and management of these complex issues; they may need support with recovery, family, daily activities, finance, general wellbeing, as well as to develop and maintain safer behaviors. By individualizing the design of care to cover all aspects of the client's needs, their potential for successfully adhering to therapy and a more positive life style can be enhanced.

REFERENCES

Ammassari, A., Trotta, M.P., Murri, R., Castelli, F., Narciso, P., Noto, P., Vecchiet, J., D'Arminio Monforte A, Wu AW, Antinori A, & AdICoNA Study Group. (2002). Correlates and Predictors of Adherence to Highly Active Antiretroviral Therapy: Overview of Published Literature. *Journal of Acquired Immune Deficiency Syndrome, 31*, Suppl 3, S123-127.

Bandura, A. (2005). The primacy of self-regulation in health promotion transformative mainstream. *Applied Psychology: An International Review, 54*, 245-254.

Bouhnik, A.D., Chesney, M., Carrieri, P., Gallais, H., Moreau, J., Moatti, J.P., Obadia, Y. Spire, B., & MANIF 2000 Study Group. (2002). Nonadherence among HIV-Infected Injecting Drug Users: The Impact of Social Instability. *Journal of Acquired Immune Deficiency Syndrome, 31* Suppl 3, S149-153.

Broadhead, R.S., Heckathorn, D.D., Altice, F.L., van Hulst, Y., Carbone, M., Friedland, G.H., O'Connor, P.G., & Selwyn, P.A. (2002) Increasing drug users' adherence to HIV treatment: Results of a peer-driven intervention feasibility study. *Social Science in Medicine, 55*(2), 235-46.

Chesney, M.A., Morin, M., & Sherr, L. (2000) Adherence to HIV Combination Therapy. *Social Science in Medicine, 50*(11), 1599-605.

Delor, F., & Hubert, M. (2000). Revisiting the concept of 'vulnerability.' *Social Science in Medicine, 50*(11), 1557-70.

Heylighen, F. (1992) A cognitive-systemic reconstruction of Maslow's theory of self-actualization. *Behavioral Science, 37*, 39-57.

Ickovics, J.R., & Meade, C.S. (2002). Adherence to HAART among patients with HIV: Breakthroughs and barriers. *AIDS Care, 14*(3), 309-318.

Ickovics, J.R., & Meade, C.S. (2002a) Adherence to Antiretroviral Therapy among Patients with HIV: A Critical Link between Behavioral and Biomedical Sciences. *Journal of Acquired Immune Deficiency Syndrome, 31*, Suppl 3, S98-102.

Paterson, D.L., Swindells, S., Mohr, J., Brester, M., Vergis, E.N., Squier, C., Wagener, M.M., & Singh N. (2000). Adherence to Protease Inhibitor Therapy and Outcomes in Patients with HIV Infection. *Annals of Internal Medicine, 133*(1), 21-30.

Sethi, A.K. Adherence and Drug Resistance. (2004). *The Hopkins HIV Report 2004, 16*(1), 7-8.

Tuldra, A., & Wu, A.W. (2002). Interventions to Improve Adherence to Antiretroviral Therapy. *Journal of Acquired Immune Deficiency Syndrome, 31*, Suppl 3, S154-157.

APPENDIX 1 Assessing the AFL: The following questions are offered as assessment suggestions to be used in conjunction with Table 1

1a. Visual cue.

1b. If client has no past history, a standard depression scale should be used.

1c. Have you ever been told that you have any medical/mental health problems? If so, have you been given any medicines to take? If yes, what do you think about that? Do you still take them? Do you think they're helping you? Are you still seeing someone about the problem that you started taking the medicine for?

1d. Do you feel that you have any kind of medical problem? If 'no' or 'don't know' and the client has a noticeable or documented problem, client is at level 1. If 'yes': Are you in treatment or do you feel that there is any medical treatment that will help? According to answer, may need to give more info and then re-question as to interest in Rx. If questioner is uncertain about need or what is his/her current treatment: defer to a medical provider for further insight as to the needs of this client (e.g., someone who acknowledges hypertension, diabetes, etc. ... but you are unclear as to how well in control the person is).

2a. A brief mental status test plus: Do you find that you have a problem remembering things?

2c. The interviewer may not be able to assess this accurately in a hospital setting until he/she has become known to and trusted by the client.

2d. Inquire where client is in care, for how long, when last appointment was and next is scheduled.

2.5a. This may be suspected from the client's responses and by inquiring into the extent of education.

2.5b. A touchy subject–if the person is Hispanic it is safe to inquire whether he/she has any difficulty reading in English? If not, and it is not apparent what their reading level is, it is safe to inquire whether he/she has any interest in improving reading skills, working toward a GED, etc.?

Reframing HIV Adherence as Part
of the Experience of Illness

Sarit A. Golub, PhD
Debbie Indyk, PhD
Milton L. Wainberg, MD

SUMMARY. Understanding and enhancing adherence to HIV medications has been identified as a major challenge. The purpose of this study was to explore patterns and determinants of non-adherence among individuals receiving HIV care in a medical clinic. Seven focus groups were conducted with 42 HIV+ patients, and verbatim transcripts of focus group sessions were analyzed through a combination of ethnographic and content analysis. Of the participants currently on combination therapy, 68% reported at least one recent instance of non-adherence. The most commonly cited reasons for non-adherent behavior were grouped into four categories: (1) problems with side effects; (2) conflicts with daily life activities; (3) feelings of aversion toward the medications themselves; and (4) deliberate alterations to the prescribed regimen.

Sarit A. Golub, PhD, is affiliated with Queens College, City University of New York. Debbie Indyk, PhD, is affiliated with Mount Sinai School of Medicine, New York, NY. Milton L. Wainberg, MD, is affiliated with the New York Psychiatric Institute, Columbia University.

Address correspondence to: Sarit A. Golub, PhD, Department of Psychology, Queens College, CUNY, 65-30 Kissena Boulevard, Flushing, NY 11367 (E-mail: sarit_golub@qc.edu).

[Haworth co-indexing entry note]: "Reframing HIV Adherence as Part of the Experience of Illness." Golub, Sarit A., Debbie Indyk, and Milton L. Wainberg. Co-published simultaneously in *Social Work in Health Care* (The Haworth Press, Inc.) Vol. 42, No. 3/4, 2006, pp. 167-188; and: *The Geometry of Care: Linking Resources, Research, and Community to Reduce Degrees of Separation Between HIV Treatment and Prevention* (ed: Debbie Indyk) The Haworth Press, Inc., 2006, pp. 167-188. Single or multiple copies of this article are available for a fee from The Haworth Document Delivery Service [1-800-HAWORTH, 9:00 a.m. - 5:00 p.m. (EST). E-mail address: docdelivery@haworthpress.com].

Available online at http://www.haworthpress.com/web/SWHC
doi:10.1300/J010v42n03_11

Findings based on structured analysis of patient responses in each category differ from past research which defines adherence as a *treatment* problem and emphasizes logistical characteristics of the treatment regimen itself and patients' ability or willingness to follow specific instructions. In contrast, our focus group data suggest an alternative frame for understanding barriers to adherence which focuses on: (1) the meaning that adherence/pill-taking behavior has for individuals experiencing chronic illness; and (2) the impact that this behavior has on their identity. Because adherence behavior is integral to patients' experience of their disease, non-adherence is no longer a *treatment* problem, but is an *illness* problem. Framing adherence as an illness problem rather than a treatment problem is a critical shift that can be applied to the creation of assessments and interventions designed to support patient adherence; this article ends with a series of specific recommendations for programs, policy, and research. *[Article copies available for a fee from The Haworth Document Delivery Service: 1-800-HAWORTH. E-mail address: <docdelivery@haworthpress.com> Website: <http://www.HaworthPress.com> © 2006 by The Haworth Press, Inc. All rights reserved.]*

KEYWORDS. Non-adherence, chronic illness, illness experience

Since combination highly active antiretroviral therapy (HAART), a treatment method designed to suppress viral replication by combining doses of at least three antiviral agents, is now the standard of care for patients with HIV infection, issues of treatment adherence have moved to the forefront of current efforts to combat the epidemic. Combination therapy is most effective only if taken *exactly* as prescribed; even minor alterations have been shown to allow the virus to develop resistance to the medications (Chesney et al., 2000; Knobel et al., 2001). Unfortunately, studies demonstrate that rates of non-adherence to HIV medications range from 15-93%, with average rates estimated to be about 50% (Chesney, 2000; Wright, 2000; Frick et al., 2001; Avants et al., 2001). The costs of such non-adherence are felt at both the individual and the societal level. For individuals, drug failure can lead to accelerated progression of the illness and limit prospects for intervention in the face of multi-drug resistant strains. For society, the emergence of resistant viral strains raises the possibility of their transmission, meaning that newly infected individuals may present for medical care with a virus that is already immune to the latest treatments. While researchers and practitioners have outlined many salient factors related to adherence, few efforts have proved successful in addressing those factors (Andrews & Freidland, 2000; Besch, 1995) or even predicting which patients will adhere to treatment and which will not (Liu et al., 2001; Bangsberg et al., 2001; Escaffre et al., 2000).

Over the last five years, over 300 articles have been cataloged in Medline related to factors that influence adherence to HIV medications. A majority of articles focus on the characteristics of the treatment regimen itself–emphasizing the complexity of regimens in terms of timing and dosage, their coordination with meal schedules and dietary restrictions, and the sheer number of pills patients are expected to take every day (Maisels, Steinberg, & Tobias, 2001; Ickovics & Meisler, 1997; Klaus & Grodesky, 1997). However, recent studies have found no association between the number of pills or dose frequency and adherence behavior (Eldred et al., 1998; Chesney, 2000). Patient characteristics such as age, gender, socioeconomic status, education and occupation have also been analyzed in terms of their impact on adherence (c.f. Kleeberger et al., 2001); but findings consistently demonstrate that these demographic characteristics are not significant predictors of whether or not the regimen is followed (Chesney et al., 2000; Ickovics & Meisler, 1997; Haynes et al., 1996; Eraker et al., 1984).

Some researchers focus on the life circumstances of HIV-patients, arguing that patients are unable to adhere because they have difficulty remembering to take their pills (Roberts & Mann, 2000), because they have cognitive limitations which make it difficult for them to understand their regimen (Avants et al., 2001), because they fail to understand or rationalize the implications of not adhering to a specific regimen (Laws, Wilson, Bowser, & Kerr, 2000), or because their lives are too hectic or chaotic to accommodate regular adherence (Klaus & Grodesky, 1997; Roberts & Mann, 2000). Other analyses have focused on patients' faith in their physicians and their belief in the efficacy of the treatment regimen, itself (Gao et al., 2000; Siegel, Karus, & Schrimshaw, 2000; Becker & Maiman, 1975) and/or the belief in the benefit of adhering to the regimen in light of debilitating and discouraging side effects which interfere with their everyday lives (Roberts & Mann, 2000).

Characteristics of the patient-provider relationship have also been analyzed to determine the extent to which this relationship contributes to patients' ability to adhere to the treatment regimen. Research suggests that the physician/patient relationship may the single most consistent factor contributing to adherence (Ickovics & Meisler, 1997). Specific patient/provider issues cited include: (a) the degree of motivation the physician demonstrates with respect to patient adherence (Waeber, Burnier, & Brunner, 2000) (b) the ability to develop a therapeutic relationship (Wright, 2000) and (c) the amount and type of communication established between the provider and the patient (Wilson & Kaplan, 2000). Recent analyses have stressed the importance of delivering culturally competent care, noting that providers' sensitivity to issues of race, ethnicity, sexual orientation, and gender identity may increase patients' willingness to seek care and adhere to treatment (Schilder et al., 2001; Kempainen et al., 2001).

More recently, researchers have begun to consider the psychological burden of adherence and are focusing on the meaning of pill-taking as HIV emerges as a chronic illness (Golub, Indyk, & Bennet, 1998; Bennet, Indyk, & Golub, 1998; Wright, 2000). For patients living with a disease that is chronic, infectious, and fatal, it is easy to imagine that the vigilance necessary to maintain their regimen can be experienced as both a blessing and a burden. In a review of factors affecting adherence, Chesney (2000) writes that the most commonly reported reasons for non-adherence are that the patient "forgot" or was "too busy" to take the medication. Such reasons are considered easily understandable and are often compared to the nearly universal experience of leaving half-filled bottles of antibiotics in the medicine cabinet after completing only some portion of a prescribed course. Without losing the empathy in communal experience that this analogy affords, it is important to recognize the difference in the meaning and psychological impact of "forgetting" when the consequence of missed doses are both dire and unforgiving, and when the pills one is "too busy" to take are toxic medications whose side effects serve as a constant reminder of both illness and treatment. Little research, if any, has placed adherence in the context of the patients' experience of illness or framed pill-taking as a behavior with psychological and emotional resonance. Such a frame is increasingly important in the context of the shifting locus of control over HIV treatment and prevention (Indyk & Golub, this volume), in which HIV-positive individuals are saddled with increased responsibility for both individual-level and public-health priorities. While providers and researchers continue to elaborate the impact on adherence of complex treatment regimens, patient-provider relationships, and other factors discussed above, it is important to utilize research methods that move beyond a mere tally of reported reasons for non-adherence toward an understanding of the motivation behind them.

The objective of this study is to use qualitative methods to explore patterns and determinants of non-adherence among individuals receiving HIV care in a medical clinic. By asking open-ended questions about adherence behavior in a focus group setting, the study was designed to allow patients to use their own words in explaining the reasons for missed doses. Through qualitative analysis of the patients' own descriptions of instances in which they did not follow their prescribed regimens, this research is intended to extend current knowledge about the meaning behind reported reasons for non-adherence and identify common themes useful in the creation of adherence assessments and interventions.

METHOD

Participants

Participants were forty-two HIV-positive patients (24 males and 18 females) of Mount Sinai Medical Center's Jack Martin Fund Clinic (JMFC), a designated AIDS Center in East Harlem, New York City. Participants ranged in age from 25 to 61, with a mean and median of 40. Demographics of the sample are reflective of the neighborhood within which the JMFC is situated, and are presented in Table 1. Thirty-five participants (87.5%) reported having taken protease inhibitors; of these, two reported starting protease inhibitors and two reported stopping protease inhibitors in the last month.

Design and Procedure

Participants attended one of seven focus groups, which ranged in size from four to eight participants each. All patients of the JMFC were eligible for participation. Study participants were recruited in the clinic waiting room using both active and passive recruitment techniques. Flyers advertising the study were placed in clinic waiting areas (passive recruitment), and a research assistant approached patients in the waiting room during randomly selected clinic sessions and asked them if they might be willing to participate (active recruitment). The active recruitment techniques were designed to reach a random sample of the clinic population; clinic sessions designated for recruitment were randomly selected and included different days and times, and the research assistant was instructed to approach every patient in the waiting room during a designated recruitment session. The combination of active and passive

TABLE 1. Participant Demographics

Variable	Number	(%)
Gender		
Male	24	(57)
Female	18	(43)
Age		
25-35	11	(27)
36-49	25	(61)
50+	5	(12)
Missing	1	
Race		
African American	17	(41)
Latino	20	(49)
White	4	(10)
Missing	1	
Marital Status		
Married/Living with someone	11	(26)
Divorced/Separated	7	(17)
Widow/er	6	(14)
Single	18	(43)
Education		
< 12 years	13	(32)
High school diploma	14	(34)
Some college	11	(27)
College degree	3	(7)
Missing	1	

techniques was designed to recruit individuals who might not volunteer for a focus group on their own (Morgan, 1990).

As part of the informed consent process, participants were told that researchers were interested in talking to them in a group setting about issues relating to adherence to HIV medications. Study staff explained that participation was voluntary and was in no way related to receipt of care at the clinic. After informed consent was obtained, participants were scheduled for a focus group session led by one of three female moderators experienced in conducting focus groups and specifically trained by the research team. Focus group questions were developed by a multidisciplinary team of HIV providers (an infectious disease specialist, a psychiatrist, a social worker, and a behavioral scientist), who reviewed the adherence literature and discussed key issues that had emerged in their own practices. The focus groups were conducted using semi-structured questionnaires consisting of open-ended questions in five areas: (1) basic questions about adherence (e.g., What is it like to take all those pills?); (2) relationship to health (e.g., Have you seen any changes in your health related to the medications?); (3) social support (e.g., How (if at all) are people in your life involved in your care?); (4) provider/patient relationship (e.g., How did you make the decision to start treatment?); and (5) health maintenance (e.g., Aside from taking your pills, are there other things you do to stay healthy?).

Because of the sensitive nature of adherence reporting, participants were assured that focus group leaders did not expect them to be 100% adherent and were reminded that any information obtained in the focus groups could not be reported to their physicians. Each focus group session lasted approximately two hours and included a 1 1/2 hour discussion, lunch, and brief pre- and post-session self-report questionnaires. Questionnaires included demographic and health status information, as well as specific questions about (i) adherence to treatment regimen; (ii) attitudes toward sexual behaviors and drug use; and (iii) the participant's personal sexual behavior and drug use. Participants were given a $15 Metrocard (transportation voucher) in appreciation of their participation. Focus group sessions were audio-taped.

Data Analysis

Verbatim transcripts of the audio-taped focus group sessions were analyzed through a combination of ethnographic and content analysis. While these two methods are often described separately, their combination–the utilization of both systematic tallying and close readings of direct quotations–is believed to enhance the strength of interpretation (Morgan, 1990). First, each specific mention of non-adherence was identified, and these instances were coded and grouped into eleven categories (see Results Section). Specific quotations within each category were then analyzed to identify trends or themes which might tie them together. As such themes were identified, the transcripts were re-coded to examine other mentions of these themes (Ely, 1993). The following results are presented in an integrative fashion designed to highlight key findings and suggest important areas for further systematic inquiry.

RESULTS

Participants' reports of their adherence behavior, both on the pre-focus group questionnaire and in the context of the focus groups, are represented in Table 2. Ten (50%) of the twenty participants who reported in the pre-focus group questionnaire that they *always* took their medication as prescribed, spoke in the focus group discussion about recent instances of non-adherence. These comments included: skipping doses, taking pills at different times or in different doses than were prescribed, and/or omitting specific medications from the regimen. In all, 27 of the 40 participants (67.5%) currently on combination therapy reported at least one instance of non-adherence.

Descriptions of each reported instance of non-adherence were coded and the reported reasons for non-adherence were group into eleven categories (Table 3). Of these, four issues emerged most frequently as the cause of non-adherent behavior: (1) problems with side effects; (2) conflicts with daily life activities; (3) feelings of aversion toward the medications themselves; and (4) deliberate alterations to the prescribed regimen. Participants also described a series of strategies that they use to help them adhere (Table 4). Participants most commonly relied on important people in their lives (partners, family members, and friends) to remind them to take their medication, but many also described using a series of reminder tools (e.g., pillbox organizers or beepers). In addition to specific instances of non-adherence, more general comments were coded to identify common themes in patients' descriptions of their experience taking the medications. Based on this analysis, two additional themes were identified as critical to understanding adherence behavior: (a) the struggle for control over both illness and treatment; and (b) the tension between feeling healthy and feeling sick.

Reasons for Non-Adherence

Problems with Side Effects. Problems with side effects was the most commonly cited reason for participants' completely discontinuing a particular drug or combination of drugs. As Paul[1] reported:

> *I stopped today . . . it's been over 30 days. It got to the point where I can't deal with the diarrhea and the headaches.*

While different participants were bothered by different types of side effects, many participants described a particular side effect that was sim-

TABLE 2. Participant Reports of Adherence Behavior in Questionnaire versus Focus Group

	Pre-Focus Group Questionnaire Number (%)	Reported Non-Adherence During Focus Group Number (%) Number (%)
Always	20 (58.8)	16 (80)
Almost always	8 (23.5)	6 (75)
Sometimes	1 (2.9)	1 (100)
Almost never	1 (2.9)	1(100)
Never	2 (5.9)	1 (50)
I have not taken protease inhibitors in the last 6 months	2 (5.9)	2 (100)
Missing	8	3 (37.5)
		30 (71% of total sample)

TABLE 3. Reasons Cited for Missing or Skipping Doses

Category	Number of Coded Responses
Can't deal with side effects	24
I'm in the middle of something	10
I just don't want to take them right now	10
I changed my own regimen	8
Too many pills	7
Forgetting	6
Can't explain to family/disclosure	4
Depression	3
Drinking/Drug Use	3
Slept through morning dose	2
Went to sleep before evening dose	2

ply intolerable to them. Once they experienced this intolerable side effect, the decision to stop the medication became clear. For example: *For me, the hardest thing to do is puke. If I'm gonna take something that's gonna make me puke, I'm not gonna do it. It's just that simple.* However, with the exception of one participant who discontinued his regimen the day of the focus group, each participant who reported stop-

TABLE 4. Strategies for Adherence

Category	Number of Coded Responses
Social support (partner, family member, friend acts as reminder)	9
Pillbox or tray	7
Beeper (including keychain, calculator, watch)	4
Calendar/time schedule	3
Alarm clock	3
Pharmacy calls or delivers	2
Associating it with other things (meals, brushing teeth)	2
Timed to the TV show schedule	1

ping a particular regimen because of side effects had resumed treatment with different medications. In addition, when side effects were alleviated or at least tolerable, they were not cited as reasons for missing individual doses or for other forms of periodic non-adherence.

Conflicts with Daily Life Activities. While side effects was most commonly cited as a reason for discontinuing therapy, the experience of missing doses "because I'm doing something," was most frequently mentioned as the reason for periodic non-adherence. Twelve individuals reported instances of this type of non-adherence; the activities in which participants were engaged during the time a given dose was scheduled included: work, school, support groups, driving, cooking dinner, sleeping, running errands, watching a ball game, playing with children, and being outside with friends. Andrew, who said that he remembered to take his medications by marking down the pills and their timing down on his calendar, reported the following:

> *Something always happens that no matter what—It's not that I forget to take them. There's always something that pops up that is more important than that.*

The distinction between forgetfulness and preoccupation, or the privileging of day-to-day activities and responsibilities as "more important" than the medication, was a recurrent theme in the focus groups. For example, Jake reported adherence problems when driving to different work appointments and explained his adherence behavior as the interaction between conscious and unconscious processes:

What I find myself doing is almost like procrastinating, but it's not. I'll say, 'OK I'll take them in an hour.' 'OK I forgot, I'll take them in an hour, unless something else comes up.' You know, and I don't . . . I do it on purpose and I don't, you know what I'm saying? When I forget it's really due to just scheduling. It's really just due to scheduling, running around.

In this brief description, Jake gives four different explanations for non-adherence that occurs in the context of daily life activities–procrastination, forgetfulness, purposeful omission, and scheduling. In most cases, the participants' descriptions of non-adherence related to daily life activities, mirrored those of Andrew and Jake; they explained that they did not *forget* their doses, but their daily activities made adherence impossible. Irene talked about her efforts to adhere in spite of her other activities:

I do a whole bunch of things–I put my alarm clock, I put another alarm clock I got there. I got the pills on me. But time passes for one reason or another and the time passed.

As will be explored in greater detail below, the process of "forgetting" doses seems active rather than passive for many of these patients. It is an action that occurs in spite of–and sometimes even in response to–memory aids designed to guard against it.

Feelings of Aversion to the Medications Themselves. Eight participants reported instances in which they missed doses because they simply did not want to take their medication. For some participants, the sheer number of pills aroused resistance. Amy and Mike described it this way:

Sometimes I get the attitude where I don't want to take it. I look at it every morning. I'm taking ten pills, then a needle at night. It really gets aggravating and depressing. (Amy)

Sometimes it's hard taking all these medicines, because sometimes you're taking ten, twelve, fifteen pills a day, and sometime you'll be like, 'I don't feel like taking all these pills. I've got to swallow all these pills.' You become a little depressed about it. (Mike)

In these instances, the number of pills in the regimen was not a barrier to adherence because patients had difficulty keeping track of their multiple medications, rather, the number of pills in the regimen presented an emotional barrier. In other instances, participants were able to identify feelings of aversion as barriers to adherence but could not articulate a clear reason behind these feelings. Linda, a 45-year-old woman who has been HIV-positive for over seven years, reported the following experience:

> *I take my medication on a regular . . . within a month I can't even think about when I've missed. I don't miss. But last night was a problem for me. At one o'clock last night I needed to take my medicine, and I was tired. I had been to a baseball game; I was totally drained when I got home. For the first time, I didn't take my medicine last night . . . so for me, being as consistent as I am, I couldn't understand what I was doing. I went like, laying in bed about 2 o'clock like, 'Now why didn't you take your medicine?' It's just that sometimes you do. I've been on protease inhibitors ever since January 1st and I never miss. Last night I was just fed up. I didn't want to take it.*

If given a quantitative checklist of reasons for non-adherence, Amy, Mike and Linda might all choose "complexity of treatment regimen"; however, their qualitative explanations of the meaning of "all these pills" indicate a more complex psychological reality. Complicated regimens are difficult to manage not only because they are physically taxing or confusing, but because they can be emotionally consuming as well.

Deliberate Alterations to the Prescribed Regimen. Finally, ten participants (24%) described a situation in which they were non-adherent because, as Christina put it, "I thought I was making my own solution," meaning that they made specific changes to their regimens in terms of medication timing, dosage, and dietary restrictions without consulting or informing their physician.

> *Instead of taking them during the day, I switched the hours to night . . . I did that on my own, because it just felt better.*

> *I kind of switched my pattern around . . . I started taking the medications an hour after drinking the methadone.*

In addition to these minor alterations, some participants had devised new regimens for themselves. Both Larry and Frank stated that they never forget their medication, but each reported a different non-adherent behavior:

> *What I do is, I'll let one day go by, like on a Sunday, I don't take no medication at all on that one particular day. [Focus Group Leader: Every Sunday?] Every Sunday. I been doing that for the longest time, just to give my body a break and stuff . . . And I find that works for me, you know, it works for me.* (Larry)

> *Now I do do one thing. I don't know whether it works or not, but once a week I omit one of my medications . . . every week I omit a different medication. Just for one day . . . I omit a different one every week, once a week.* (Frank)

These examples belie the assumption that patients have trouble with adherence because regimens are too difficult to follow; in some cases, the regimens that patients devised for themselves were even more complicated than those they had been prescribed. While deliberate alterations to the treatment regimen seems to be a different type of reason for non-adherence than side-effects, conflicts with daily life activities, or feelings of aversion to medications, all four categories come together to elaborate the meaning of non-adherence in the context of participants' struggle to live with chronic illness.

Emergent Themes in Participant's Discussions of Adherence

Struggle for Control over both Illness and Treatment. In addition to describing specific instances of non-adherence, participants discussed adherence in the context of other over-arching issues. Participants talked about having more control over their illness as a result of combination therapy, and in some instances, the act of pill-taking/adherence itself was described as a form of disease management.

> *I believe I'm doing better from taking the meds . . . it's just the idea of knowing, for me, that I'm doing something about my condition.*

> *When I miss my pills I feel guilty. I feel like I'm not doing it directly for myself, so I always try to take my medication. I feel every time I put it in my mouth it's killing the virus. That's how I look at it.*

At the same time, participants also discussed the fact that their new sense of control over their illness and treatment came with a corresponding dependence on the medications themselves. As David put it:

> *You feel good, you look good, you're on top of the world. But how you get there, that's the most important thing to remember, and the way to stay on top of the world is to continue taking the medications.*

In addition, many participants articulated a tension over which member of the treatment team–the doctor or the patient–was in control of the treatment regimen and responsible for the successes engendered by it. Larry described the creation of his current treatment plan this way:

> *When the protease inhibitors came by, my doctor wanted to find out which were the ones that would really work for me. I had to try several different ones before I really, before they could really find out which ones worked for me.* [emphasis added]

Steve explained that instead of "stressing" about a particular regimen, he took his pills whenever he woke up in the morning:

> *See, you have to start doing it your own way. The doctors will tell you a way, but you have to do it the way that will be better for you.*

Feeling Healthy and Feeling Sick. Thirteen focus group participants (30%) talked about how much healthier they felt after starting new medication regimens. Eva explained that before she started taking protease inhibitors, she had been given only six months to live:

> *I came down with progressive multi-focal encephalopathy, which is always fatal, and it affects your spinal cord system and your brain . . . then, when I went on the protease, I just . . . [participant snaps]. I was in a wheelchair, I just got up and started running.*

Other patients reported similar improvements and credited their adherence to treatment regimens with transforming their lives. However, participants also talked about how sick the medications made them feel.

> *Before I was feeling good, and when I started taking the medication I was bedridden. I was sick, sick, totally sick.*

> *It [the medication] might help viral load or the CD-count. It might do all that, but you be so sick getting there.*

In addition to identifying physical side effects, the participants explained that the medications made them feel sick by serving as constant reminders of their illness. As Jake and David explained:

> *For me, what it was is like a beautiful day like today. I'd get up in the morning, and here are these pills to remind me I'm sick. And I just didn't want to think that way.* (Jake)

> *Before 1990, I remember myself as being one very healthy person . . . I never had to take any kind of medications. Now I have to, I have to take them on a daily basis . . . if I'm outside and I'm doing something and I'm enjoying myself, I know that I gotta go home and take the medication.* (David)

DISCUSSION

Each of the specific categories related to non-adherent behavior–problems with side effects, conflicts with daily life activities, feelings of aversion to medications themselves, and deliberate alterations to the treatment regimen–raise important issues for the assessment and support of adherence among patients receiving treatment in a clinic setting. Each category represents an important component of the determinant of adherence behavior, and specific interventions can be developed and tested relating to these issues.

Participants' comments about their conflicting feelings of control over their medications and illness are consistent with past research on other chronic illnesses and disability. The onset of chronic, life-threatening illness has been found to be accompanied by a loss of personal control (Fife, 1994; Karp, 1994), and adaptation to chronic illness has been described in terms of a tension between feelings of competence and helplessness (Viney & Westbrook, 1981; Alexander, 1976). For HIV-positive individuals, adherence to treatment regimens exemplifies this tension between dependence and independence. If they adhere to these regimens, patients become more independent; they feel better, their clinical symptoms improve, and they need less acute care. However, adherence is also associated with a corresponding dependence on the medications themselves and on regimens controlled by medical providers. Seen in this light, non-adherence due to deliberate alterations in treatment regimens may stem not from patients' lack of ability or willingness to follow their prescribed regimen, but out of a desire to assert their own agency. Active participation in the determination of their treatment regimen–contributing to the discovery of a regimen that "works for me"–may foster a sense of personal control over an illness that seems to be controlled only by medication.

The tension between feeling healthy and feeling sick has been identified by many researchers as part of the assimilation of chronic illness or disability into an individual's self-concept (Mechanic, 1995; Antonak & Livneh, 1985). Since illness often implies deviance from social conceptions of healthy or "normal" behavior and experience (Karp, 1994), chronic illness can pose a significant challenge to an individual's identity, especially if the disease is life-threatening. Similar to its impact on feelings of dependence and independence, adherence to HIV medication simultaneously supports the infected individuals' view of themselves as both "healthy" and "sick." While new medications have helped HIV-positive individuals feel much healthier, they also serve as constant reminders that HIV-infected individuals are still "sick." While few patients articulate the assimilation of illness into their identity as a specific barrier to adherence, reports of particular instances of non-adherence under each category–problems with side effects, conflicts with daily life activities, feelings of aversion toward the medications themselves, and conscious decisions to alter the regimen–make sense in terms of patients' desire not to feel "sick." Participants who stopped taking pills because of side effects spoke about how "sick" the medication made them feel. In contrast, the one individual who stayed on his medication in spite of side effects said that he was able to continue with the medications because he believed it would keep him from getting sick.

Adherence problems due to conflicts with daily life activities can also be seen as resistance to constant reminders of illness, especially when pill taking interrupts moments in which patients are feeling particularly healthy or normal. This interpretation of conflicts with daily life activities as related to patients' self-concept might explain why participants reported that their efforts to use beepers or other reminder devices did not help them adhere. Andrew's explanation that something always "pops up" that is "more important" than the medication may be an expression of what living the life of a healthy person means to him–daily activities are more important than pills. It also sheds some light on Jake's conflicted account of his non-adherence as both purposeful and accidental; he may not want to remind himself of his illness while performing pre-HIV activities such as working and driving.

Instances in which patients reported feelings of aversion to pills themselves may be even clearer examples of resistance to constant reminders of illness. Linda described her first act of non-adherence after spending the day at a ball game; perhaps after engaging in an activity that made her feel particularly healthy or "normal," she did not want to engage in a behavior that would characterize her as a sick person. The sheer number of pills patients have to take may be "depressing" in and of themselves because pill taking is associated with serious illness.

The large number of patients from minority groups in the study sample merits some attention in light of conflicting views regarding the role of ethnicity as a determining factor in adherence behavior. As noted above, several studies have found lower rates of adherence to HIV medications among non-white populations (Singh et al., 1996; Muma et al., 1995; Kleeberger, 2001). However, other studies of adherence behavior both among HIV positive patients and among patients with other diseases have generated mixed findings about the relationship between adherence and race (Ickovics & Meisler, 1997; Besch, 1995; Morgan, 1995; Hellman et al., 1997), and a report from the Forum for Collaborative HIV Research (1998) stated that demographic characteristics including race are not significant predictors of adherence. It is disturbing, therefore, that some research suggests that attitudes about non-white patients' potential for adherence influence providers decisions about starting them on therapy (Bogart, 2001). While the sample size and racial distribution in this study make it difficult to draw definitive conclusions about racial or gender differences, the psychological issues that emerged were remarkably similar across all participants. However, since interventions focusing on the meaning of adherent and non-adherent behavior must necessarily reflect differences in patients' relationship with the health care system and health care providers, further research and attention is needed into the racial, ethnic, and gender differences in the experience of illness and treatment.

Finally, while focus groups serve as a valuable tool in understanding the adherence experiences of HIV-positive patients, there are some limitations inherent in the methodology. First, most focus groups, including the ones in this study, are composed of convenience samples; individuals willing to discuss the experiences in a group setting may not necessarily be representative of the entire population (Kirk & Miller, 1986). Second, focus group discussions are profoundly influenced by group dynamics and have the potential to both under- and over-represent experiences of participants (Ely, 1993). Given this potential, tabulations of participant comments should be looked at merely as a summary of the coding process; themes arise because of their analytic impact and may be equally valid regardless of frequency (Ely, 1993). However, the strengths of focus groups lie in their ability to shed light on participants' experiences and perspectives, and in their explicit use of group interaction to produce data and insights that would be less accessible through another medium (Morgan, 1990).

IMPLICATIONS FOR PRACTICE

In most current discussions of adherence to HIV medications, barriers to adherence are construed in terms of: (1) logistical characteristics of the treatment regimen itself and its complex and demanding nature; and (2) the patient's ability or willingness to follow specific instructions due to memory problems, cognitive limitations, or chaotic life-circumstances (Forum for Collaborative HIV Research et al., 1998). In these analyses, non-adherence is framed as a *treatment* problem and barriers to adherence are construed in terms of the patient's experience of the medication regimen itself. As a result, strategies to enhance adherence have also focused on the treatment regimen. Patients are given beepers, medication calendars, pill organizers, improved educational materials and case management to improve adherence (Ickovics & Meisler, 1997; Bond & Hussar, 1991).

Framing adherence as a *treatment* problem forces a distinction between the experience of treatment and the experience of illness. Researchers talk about the costs of *non-adherence* in terms of illness, relapse and recovery (Ickovics & Meisler, 1997), but few talk about the costs of *adherence* to the patient in terms of quality of life and identity. For individuals with an acute, curable disease, it may be possible to separate the experience of treatment from the experience of illness, because treatment becomes part of the process of recovery. For HIV-positive individuals, treatment cannot be associated with total recovery but instead, becomes part of the process of living with illness.

While treatment-related barriers were mentioned by participants, the above focus group data suggests an alternative frame for understanding adherence which focuses on: (1) the meaning that adherence/pill-taking behavior has for individuals experiencing chronic illness; and (2) the impact that this behavior has on their identity. When adherence is described as a treatment problem, it is traditionally defined as "the extent to which a person's behavior conforms with medical or health advice" (Besch, 1995). In the above analysis, patients' instances of non-adherence–because of problems with side effects, conflicts with daily life activities, feelings of aversion to the medications themselves, or conscious decisions to alter the regimen–were less a result of difficulties conforming to medical advice, and more strongly related to difficulties with the experience and meaning of taking pills–the conflict between feeling competent or helpless and between feeling healthy or sick. Because adherence behavior is integral to patients' experience of their illness, non-adherence is not only a *treatment* problem, it is an *illness* problem as well. Framing adherence as an *illness* problem acknowledges that pill-taking behavior–and indeed, all aspects of self-management of chronic illness–takes place within the context of an individual's illness experience.

Reframing adherence as an *illness* problem is a call for future research, not only to further elaborate the issues and barriers to adherence, but also to identify the structural changes and professional training needs necessary to address them. In the same way that researchers now use convergent methods to assess adherence behavior (e.g., self-report, pill count, MEMs caps), multiple methods must also be used to understand the reasons behind this behavior. Specifically, future research should consider adherence behavior in light of the psychological demands inherent in coping with chronic illness. In shaping a research agenda, it might prove useful to focus on the patients who *are* adherent, identifying the ways in which they have been able to integrate pill-taking and other health-maintenance behaviors into their lives and experience of illness. For practitioners, framing adherence as an illness problem means recognizing the impact of both illness and treatment on a patient's life and personal identity. Adherence support and interventions would then extend beyond mnemonic devices to include counseling, buddy programs, and support groups. If strategies to assess and enhance adherence to HIV treatment regimens begin framing the problem in terms of patients' experience with illness, future efforts may prove extremely successful in improving patient adherence and combating future morbidity and mortality associated with the epidemic.

NOTE

1. All names are pseudonyms.

REFERENCES

Alexander, L. (1976). The double-bind theory and hemodialysis. *Archives of General Psychiatry*, *33*, 1351-1356.

Andrews, L., & Friedland, G. (2000). Progress in HIV therapeutics and the challenges of adherence to antiretroviral therapy. *Infectious Disease Clinics of North America*, *14*(4): 910-28.

Antonak, R.F., & Livneh, H. (1985). Psychosocial adaptation to disability and its investigation among persons with multiple sclerosis. *Social Science and Medicine*, *40*, 1099-1108.

Avants, S.K., Margolin, A., Warburton, L.A., Hawkins, K.A., & Shi, J. (2001). Predictors of nonadherence to HIV-related medication regimens during methadone stabilization. *American Journal of Addiction*, *10*(1): 69-78.

Bangsberg, D.R., Hecht, F.M., Clague, H., Charlebois, E.D., Ciccarone, D., Chesney, M., & Moss, A. (2001). Provider assessment of adherence to HIV antiretroviral therapy. *Journal of Acquired Immune Deficiency Syndrome*, *26*(5): 435-42.

Becker, M.H., & Maiman, L.A. (1975) Sociobehavioral determinants of compliance with health and medical care recommendations. *Medical Care*, *13*(1), 10-24.

Bennett, M., Indyk, D., & Golub, S. (1998). Adherence re-framed in the BIG picture: A qualitative ecological perspective on HIV+ patients and protease inhibitors. In: Programs and abstracts of the 12th World AIDS Conference. Geneva: Marathon Multimedia.

Besch, C.L. (1995). Compliance in clinical trials. *AIDS*, *9*(1), 1-10.

Bogart, L.M., Catz, S.L., Kelly, J.A., & Benotsch, E.G. (2001). Factors influencing physicians' judgments of adherence and treatment decisions for patients with HIV disease. *Medical Decision Making*, *21*(1): 28-36.

Bond, W.S., & Hussar, D.A. (1991). Detection methods and strategies for improving medication compliance. *American Journal of Hospital Pharmacology*, *48*(9), 1978-88.

Chesney, M. (2000). Factors affecting adherence to antiretroviral therapy. *Clinical Infectious Diseases*, *30*(S2):S171-176.

Chesney, M.A., Morin, M., & Sherr, L. (2000). Adherence to HIV combination therapy. *Social Science & Medicine, 50(11)*, 1599-1605.

Cresop-Fierro, M. (1997). Compliance/adherence and care management in HIV disease. *Journal of the Association of Nurses in AIDS Care*, *8*(4), 43-54.

Easterbrook, P.J., Keruly, J.C., Creagh-Kirk, T., Richman, D.D., Chaisson, R.E., & Moore, R.D. The Zidovudine Epidemiology Study Group. (1991). Racial and ethnic differences in outcome in zidovudine-treated patients with advanced HIV disease. *Journal of the American Medical Association*, *266*(19), 2713-2718.

Eldred, L.J., WU, A.W., Chaisson, R.E., & Moore, R.D. (1998). Adherence to antiretroviral and pneumocystis prophylaxis in HIV disease. *Journal of Acquired Immune Deficiency Syndrome Retrovirology*, *18*: 117-25.

Ely, M. (1993) *Doing qualitative research: Circles within circles*. Bristol, PA: Falmer.

Eraker, S.A., Kirscht, J.P., & Becker, M.H. (1984). Understanding and improving patient compliance. *Annals of Internal Medicine*, *100*, 258-268.

Escaffre, N., Morin, M., Bouhnil, A.D., Fuzibet, J.G., Gastaut, J.A., Obadia, Y., Moatti, J.P., Manif 2000 Study Group. Injecting drug users adherence to HIV antiretroviral treatments: Physician's beliefs. *AIDS Care, 12*(6): 723-30.

Fife, B.L. (1994). The conceptualization of meaning in illness. *Social Science and Medicine, 38*(2), 309-316.

Forum for Collaborative HIV Research, National Minority AIDS Council, & National Institutes of Health Office of AIDS Research. (1998). Understanding adherence. *Proceedings of Adherence to New HIV Therapies: A Research Conference.* Washington, DC: Author.

Frick, P.A., Lavreys, L., Mandaliya, K., & Kreiss, J.K. (2001). Impact of an alarm device on medication compliance in women in Mombasa, Kenya. *International Journal of STD and AIDS, 12*(5): 329-33.

Gao, X., Nau, D.P., Rosenbluth, S.A., Scott, V., & Woodward, C. (2000). The relationship of disease severity, health beliefs and medication adherence among HIV patients. *AIDS Care, 12*(4): 387-98.

Golub, S., Indyk, D.I., & Bennett, M. (1998, November). Reframing adherence to HIV medication regimens. Presented at the *American Public Health Association* annual meeting, Washington D.C.

Haynes, R.B., Mckibbon, K.A., & Kanani, R. (1996) Systematic review of randomized trials of interventions to assist patient to follow prescriptions for medications. *Lancet, 348*(9024), 383-86.

Hellman, S., Baker, L., Flores, D., Lehman, H., & Bacon, J. (1997). The effect of ethnicity on adherence to diabetic regimen. *Ethnicity and Disease, 7*(3), 221-8.

Ickovics, J.R., & Meisler, A.W. (1997). Adherence in AIDS clinical trials: A framework for clinical research and clinical care. *Journal of Clinical Epidemiology, 50*(4), 385-391.

Karp, D.A. (1994). Living with depression: Illness and identity turning points. *Qualitative Health Research, 4*(1):6-30.

Kemppainen, J.K., Leving, R.E., Mistal, M., & Schmidgall, D. (2001). HARRT adherence in culturally diverse patients with HIV/AIDS: As study of male patients from a Veteran's Administration Hospital in northern California. *AIDS Patient Care and STDS, 15*(3): 117-27.

Kirk, J., & Miller, M.L. *Reliability and validity in qualitative research.* Beverly Hills, CA: Sage.

Klaus, B.D., & Grodesky, M.J. (1997). Assessing and enhancing compliance with antiretroviral therapy. *Nurse Practitioner, 22*(4), 211-216.

Kleeberger, C.A., Phair, J.P, Strathdee, S.A., Detels, R., Kingsley, L., & Jacobson, L.P. (2001). Determinants of heterogeneous adherence to HIV-antiretroviral therapies in the Multicenter AIDS Cohort Study. *Journal of Acquired Immune Deficiency Syndrome, 26*(1): 82-92.

Knobel, H., Guelar, A., Carmona, A., Espona, M., Gonzalez, A., Lopez-Colomes, J.L., Saballs, P., Gimeno, J.L., & Diez, A. (2001). Virologic outcome and predictors of virologic failure of highly active antiretroviral therapy containing protease inhibitors. *AIDS Patient Care STDS, 15*(4): 193-199.

Laws, M.B., Wilson, I.B., Bowser, D.M., & Kerr, S.E. (2000). Taking antiretroviral therapy for HIV infection: Learning from patients' stories. *Journal of General Internal Medicine, 15*(12):848-58.

Liu, H., Golin, C.E., Miller, L.G., Hays, R.D., Beck, C.K., Sanandaji, S., Christian, J., Maldonado, T., Duran, D. Kaplan, A.H., & Wenger, N.S. (2001). A comparison study of multiple measures of adherence to HIV protease inhibitors. *Annals of Internal Medicine, 134*(10): 968-77.

Maisels, L., Steinberg, J., & Tobias, C. (2001) An investigation of why eligible patients do not receive HAART. *AIDS Patient Care and STDS, 15*(4): 185-91.

Mangus, M., Schmidt, N., Kirkhart, K., Schieffelin, C., Fuchs, N., Brown, B., & Kissinger, P.J. (2001). Association between ancillary services and clinical and behavioral outcomes among HIV-infected women. *AIDS Patient Care and STDS, 15*(3): 137-45.

Mechanic, D.M. (1995). Sociological dimensions of illness behavior. *Social Science and Medicine, 41*(9), 1207-1216.

Morgan, D.L. (1990). *Focus Groups as Qualitative Research.* Newbury Park, CA: Sage.

Morgan, M. (1995). The significance of ethnicity for health promotion: Patients' use of anti-hypertensive drugs in inner London. *International Journal of Epidemiology, 24*(Suppl. 1), S79-S84.

Muma, R.D., Ross, M.W., Parcel, G.S., & Pollard, R.B. (1995). Zidovudine adherence among individuals with HIV infection. *AIDS Care, 7*(4): 439-47.

Roberts, K.J., & Mann, T. (2000). Barriers to antiretroviral medication adherence in HIV-infected women. *AIDS Care, 12*(4): 377-86.

Schilder, A.J., Kennedy, C., Goldstone, I.L., Ogden, R.D., Hogg, R.S., & O'Shaughnessy, M.V. (2001). "Being dealt with as a whole person." Care seeking and adherence: The benefits of culturally competent care. *Social Science and Medicine, 52*(11): 1643-59.

Siegel, K., Karus, D., & Schrimshaw, E.W. (2000). Racial differences in attitudes toward protease inhibitors among older HIV-infected men. *AIDS Care, 12*(4): 423-34.

Singh, N., Squier, C, Sivek, C., Wagener, M., Nguyen, M.H., & Yu, V.L. (1996). Determinants of compliance with antiretroviral therapy in patients with human immunodeficiency virus: Prospective assessment with implications for enhancing compliance. *AIDS Care, 8*(3): 261-269.

Stephenson, B.J. (1993). Is the patient taking the treatment as prescribed? *Journal of the American Medical Association, 269*(21), 2779-2781.

Viney, L.L., & Westbrook, M.T. (1981). Psychological reactions to chronic illness-related disability as a function of its severity and type. *Journal of Psychosomatic Research, 25*(6), 513-523.

Waeber, B., Burnier, M., & Brunner, H.R. (2000). How to improve adherence with prescribed treatment in hypertensive patients? *Journal of Cardiovascular Pharmacology, 35*: S23-S26.

Wilson, I.B., & Kaplan, S. (2000). Physician-patient communication in HIV disease: The importance of patient, physician, and visit characteristics. *Journal of Acquired Immune Deficiency Syndrome, 25*(5):417-25.

Wright, M.T. (2000). The old problem of adherence: Research on treatment adherence and its relevance for HIV/AIDS. *AIDS Care, 12*(6): 703-710.

Pediatric HIV Adherence:
An Ever-Evolving Challenge

Jocelyn Childs, LCSW
Nancy Cincotta, LCSW

SUMMARY. Providers working with children living with HIV strive to achieve "good adherence," often viewed only as consistent pill taking by the infected child. This goal, while important, needs to be expanded with a thorough examination of the many biopsychosocial factors impacting the HIV affected family. The complexity of the issues affecting adherence to a pediatric HIV medical regimen can overwhelm both the practitioner and the patient. By utilizing a developmental framework and emphasizing the critical importance of the relationship between provider, patient and family, the authors (both of whom are social workers who have worked over a period of many years with children and families living with terminal and serious chronic illnesses) describe a developmental approach that includes comprehensive assessment to address the multiple challenges faced by individuals and families they have worked with. *[Article copies available for a fee from The Haworth Document Delivery Service: 1-800-HAWORTH. E-mail address: <docdelivery@haworthpress.com> Website: <http://www.HaworthPress.com> © 2006 by The Haworth Press, Inc. All rights reserved.]*

Jocelyn Childs, LCSW, and Nancy Cincotta, LCSW, are affiliated with Mount Sinai Medical Center, New York, NY.

[Haworth co-indexing entry note]: "Pediatric HIV Adherence: An Ever-Evolving Challenge." Childs, Jocelyn, and Nancy Cincotta. Co-published simultaneously in *Social Work in Health Care* (The Haworth Press, Inc.) Vol. 42, No. 3/4, 2006, pp. 189-208; and: *The Geometry of Care: Linking Resources, Research, and Community to Reduce Degrees of Separation Between HIV Treatment and Prevention* (ed: Debbie Indyk) The Haworth Social Work Practice Press, an imprint of The Haworth Press, Inc., 2006, pp. 189-208. Single or multiple copies of this article are available for a fee from The Haworth Document Delivery Service [1-800-HAWORTH, 9:00 a.m. - 5:00 p.m. (EST). E-mail address: docdelivery@haworthpress.com].

KEYWORDS. Pediatric AIDS, family-centered social work, disclosure, child development

Adherence to the medical regimen has been noted to be the major determinant of the success of HAART–Highly Active Antiretroviral Therapy (Watson et al., 1999) and plays a critical role in the treatment of the HIV+ child (Stone, 2001). Assessment and detailed examination of adherence are made difficult by its idiosyncratic nature, and by a lack of complete understanding of the challenges to adherence for the HIV+ patient. While it is readily acknowledged that HIV adherence in adults is multi-determined (Fogarty et al., 2002), the variables affecting a child's adherence are considerably greater given the complex nature of factors and systems involved in the treatment of a child.

Extrapolating purely pediatric adherence issues from the broader spectrum of HIV adherence is challenging since HIV is a family disease. In families affected by HIV there is often more than one family member who is ill, and the sequelae of each individual's illness affects each family member differently; this matrix of factors affects the child's adherence.

Both the new geometry of care (Rier & Indyk, this volume) and the shifting locus of HIV treatment and prevention (Indyk & Golub, this volume) have critical implications for issues surrounding pediatric adherence. Children cannot be seen as existing outside the context of their families. HIV typically affects the most disenfranchised of families: those overwhelmed by illness, poverty, substance abuse, mental illness and homelessness (Weiner et al., 1992). Children are at the same disadvantage as adults in terms of having complex, interconnected psychosocial issues that affect their own, and their family members' ability to cope, nonetheless adhere to a treatment regimen. Compounding the challenges that are faced by most adults with HIV are the children's own unique and ever-changing developmental conceptions of health and illness, as well as their cognitive abilities. The challenge for practitioners is how to assess and address the personal, cognitive, developmental, familial and social factors that affect a child's adherence to HIV medications.

The unique characteristics of the HIV virus require taking all antiretrovirals with near perfect adherence (Friedland & Williams, 1999) to prevent the development of resistant virus (Patterson, 2000). Improved health outcomes for children are dependent upon maximum viral suppression, which is a result of consistent adherence. While taking medications in a regimented manner is the ultimate goal of adherence, it is important to contextualize adherence in terms of a hierarchy of tasks necessary to reach this goal. Accessing medical care, obtaining appropriate treatment, having the ability to openly discuss potential barriers to adherence with medical providers, and working in a trusting relationship with the medical team are some of the prerequisites to adherence. In the case of pediatric HIV, a parallel structure of assessment, both of the needs and capabilities of the child and the adult caregiver, is required.

DEVELOPMENT CHALLENGES AND CONSIDERATIONS

The process of adherence is not static, but is constantly being affected by external factors. One of the greatest challenges in assessing and addressing pediatric adherence is that as the child develops, the barriers to adherence change. In children, developmental changes may seem apparent, but without an actual assessment of the child's HIV knowledge, understanding of why they take medications, feelings, reactions and coping style, the clinician may not have adequate knowledge of the child's ability to comprehend (emotionally and cognitively), nonetheless adhere to a regimen. When caretakers perceive they have tackled one challenge successfully, they may become frustrated, because as the child matures, new concerns arise. Generally, increased age can be associated with greater knowledge about HIV and the concomitant medication regimen. However, greater knowledge can bring with it more complicated emotional responses, which can positively or negatively affect the ability to adhere. We describe below various stage specific developmental challenges and considerations based on examples from our practice to demonstrate the dynamic adherence issues confronting caregivers and children living with HIV.

Newborns, Infants and Toddlers. Often parents of a newborn appear to either suppress or deny their anxiety about the illness. This coping strategy, though somewhat effective during pregnancy, becomes less adaptive once the child is born. The reality of the baby and the concrete tasks of caring for that baby bring uncomfortable emotions into consciousness. The arrival of the baby is supposed to be an exciting time. There are appropriate feelings of grief and loss when processing a child's exposure to HIV, which require time to adjust to. Yet, any ambivalence a parent may feel about the child because of HIV could heighten a personal sense of inadequacy. In addition, the parent may feel that there will be a societal perception that the parent's uncertainty reflects poor parenting. These conflicts make it difficult to openly discuss the parent's reaction to the illness and her ability to take care of the child. The challenges faced by parents are normal, but many a new mother is under the illusion that she should be able to easily cope with, confront and eradicate any difficulty, including HIV. Therefore, anxiety about the medication, either due to concerns about its efficacy or frustrations with its administration, is usually a taboo topic for discussion from the point of view of new parents.

> *Parents have talked about feeling coerced by providers–that if they didn't give the medications they would be deemed poor parents and that their child would be taken away. One parent was able to share, after much support, that initially she had thought it would be best to give up her child to ACS. Rather than make a mistake with the medication and be held responsible by the providers, she felt she should preemptively punish herself, her fear of the consequences of non-adherence was so great.*

Parents of newborns are also faced with their own guilt and blame because of the transmission of HIV to the newborn. These feelings, compounded with the range of emotions experienced after a birth, may further compromise a parent's ability to immediately adhere to an aggressive treatment regimen for the child.

> *One mother said she was so overwhelmed by the fear that her baby was going to become HIV+ that her anxiety kept her up all night. She became so distraught and sleepless that she ultimately missed giving her baby medication doses due to sheer fatigue. Her mind was so "consumed with guilt" and anxiety that she had little energy to focus on any form of prevention.*

Administering the medications to an infant is relatively straightforward, yet creating a schedule can be difficult. Some of the medications need to be given on an empty stomach. For a baby who feeds every few hours, how does one easily find a time when the baby has not just eaten and is awake (Hutton, 2003)? Caregivers may also feel anxious about giving such potent medications to a small baby, particularly if they themselves have experienced adverse effects from the same or similar medications.

While it may be the standard of care to give AZT to all newborns exposed to HIV, to a parent who believes their child will be disease-free, giving such a powerful substance to an infant can seem counter-intuitive.

> *Eventually, one mother, was able to share her concern that as the virus was being killed by the medication, she thought it was also killing her baby. Another mother talked about her fear of giving AZT to her newborn when it wasn't yet determined whether or not her son was actually infected with the virus. "I've already hurt him enough (by exposing him to HIV)–these medicines may do him in."*

As the baby gets older and becomes more mobile, the issues seem to grow and change. The quantity of medication increases as the child gains weight and the amount the child needs to consume can seem daunting. The tastes of the liquid medications are often difficult to mask. Most adults, after tasting some of the medications, find that they have a newfound respect for the children who manage to tolerate them. In addition, the number of medications necessary (even for an infant) can make the administration of a HAART regimen extremely difficult (Goode, 2003).

> *One father described his daily confusion about the numerous medications. Trying to remember which syringe went with which medication, which medication addressed which concern and when to administer them was taxing.*

Toddlers, as they begin to search for a sense of autonomy, typically become defiant. It can be very demanding on a caregiver to battle the child to take his medication. It may take hours for a child to actually finish a single dose of the medications.

> *Parents have called, crying in frustration. The time, the patience and the energy needed to struggle with a toddler taking medication are often difficult to find. A common complaint is that by the time the child has finished taking one dose it is time to begin with the next.*

Preschool and School Age Children. While an older child can go through the process of learning how to swallow pills, this does not elim-

inate the challenge. HIV medications are formulated for the adult patient. For all children, the size of the pills can be overwhelming.

> *One child was tremendously proud after many sessions of 'pill tak-*
> *ing classes' when she accomplished the goal of learning how to*
> *swallow all her pills. Unfortunately, soon after her regimen was*
> *altered, and her new medications were only dispensed in pills*
> *twice the size of the ones she had practiced with. Her sense of de-*
> *feat was disheartening.*

When the child enters school other barriers emerge. If a parent
chooses not to disclose the child's HIV status to the school and the child
is on medications many times a day, some doses may be skipped. As a
result, physicians have to alter regimens to include only medications
that can be given twice a day, thereby avoiding this dilemma (Byrne,
2002). This has evolved to be a less common phenomenon as pharmaceutical companies have formulated many of the medications to be
taken twice a day, yet for some children this remains an issue.

Children of school age want to be like their peers. When they learn
that no one else has to take medications, the daily pills are a constant reminder to the HIV+ children that they are indeed different, and that they
have to deal with an illness that no one else has to contend with.

> *These children are quick to acknowledge that their burden is "un-*
> *fair." And it is. "Every day it is like someone is telling me again*
> *that there is something wrong with me. I might be able to forget*
> *that, if I didn't have to take the pills."*

This dynamic is further complicated by the fact that no one at school
may know the child's diagnosis. Children often need the support, encouragement and surveillance of an adult to take medications and to
cope with other illness-related issues that may emerge.

> *One parent disclosed her child's HIV diagnosis to the school so*
> *the nurse could help administer the medication and provide sup-*
> *port in case of an emergency. The disclosure had the reverse effect*
> *of support. Each time the child coughed, sneezed or got a bruise,*
> *she would be sent home from school. The school's anxiety and ig-*
> *norance about the disease only served to complicate the child's*
> *life and her adherence. It was easier when the school did not know.*

Unfortunately, the message supported the concept that secrecy is the best policy.

Disclosure, while an issue for a child of any age, becomes paramount as a child's cognitive abilities develop. Many younger children do not know their diagnosis. It is difficult to stress adherence when they have an incomplete understanding of their illness and limited awareness of the consequences of non-adherence. When children do not understand what is going on inside their bodies, they have a difficult time recognizing the benefits of the medications on their immune system.

Children of school age who do not know their diagnosis frequently question providers about the medication. Their questions are justified and unfortunately without disclosure, the answers they get from family and staff do not necessarily serve to inform them, reassure them, or make them more likely to be adherent. One mother's attempt to explain HIV metaphorically as "monsters in the blood" caused more nightmares than comfort.

Disclosure, however, doesn't guarantee adherence. For many children, knowing their diagnosis may actually complicate matters. For a child who has had family members die from AIDS, there may be a strong sense of survival guilt combined with a fear that a parent's death is a predictor of his or her own future. The array of emotional conflicts facing children of the epidemic may serve to complicate their feelings regarding adherence.

A child who was the one survivor (her mother, father, grandmother and sister all died of AIDS) expressed not only an ambivalence towards life (she had some desire to join her family) but a sense of herself as 'different,' not a positive sense. It seemed she felt that there was something wrong with her as she survived this disease that had taken away everyone that she loved.

During the latency period (approximately 5-12 years of age), children are particularly sensitive to issues of health and illness as they come to understand the irreversibility and inevitability of death (Speece & and Brent, 1984). Typically it is the symptoms of illness that are the focus of anxiety (Cincotta, 2002). For a child with HIV, where there are not apparent outward signs of illness, the medication may become the focus of their concern. To avoid uncomfortable feelings or feeling different from everyone else, children, even at young ages, may not take their medications. Some children will use extreme measures to hide their medications and pretend they were consumed.

> *One parent was cleaning her couch where she found over three month's worth of medication that the child had not swallowed.*

When children's understanding of their illness is vague, they will create their own interpretation of what is going on. Often the fantasy is worse than reality (Cincotta, 2004), which is another reason to encourage open communication regarding HIV.

> *Many teens, as they reflect back to earlier years when they learned their diagnosis, have described the relief they felt. One remembered her mother's shock when her comment was, "Is that all?" to the disclosure of HIV. HIV was normative and chronic in her eyes; she had worried that she had cancer of her stomach and was afraid each day it was slowly eating away at her.*

Even under the optimal circumstance when a child knows her HIV status and has a good understanding of her illness, there may be other family members who are unaware of the diagnosis. Quite often the parent and child may spend an exorbitant amount of time and emotional energy maintaining this family secret. Relabelling bottles, finding hiding places for the medications, and creating elaborate scenarios to keep people from questioning the child's health, all take their toll on the child, the parent and the adherence process.

> *One mother shared her confusion that would result from the process of hiding the diagnosis. She would have to pick up the medicines from the pharmacy (home delivery was out of the question as the pills could fall into the wrong hands) buy new labels to concoct an asthma diagnosis for her child, and store them in hiding places all over the apartment. In all of these efforts she would forget the real dosages of medication and often misplace the real bottles.*

The burden of keeping the secret of HIV can be detrimental to the child's emotional well being. Children can quickly develop an unspoken sense of shame about HIV and their own bodies (Sherman et al., 2000; Weiner et al., 1993) when the message they are given is "to keep this information 'secret' or 'private.'" These feelings can easily be projected onto the medications and affect the child's ability to adhere.

Throughout most of childhood, thought processes remain concrete (Ginsburg and Opper, 1998). It makes sense for a child to think, *"Why should I have to take medicines when I feel good?"* or, *"When I take the medications I feel bad, so I should stop taking them."* A thorough, ongoing assessment of the child's perception and understanding of HIV is critical. As children's cognitive abilities increase, the information imparted to them needs to be readjusted and expanded (Cincotta, 1993). With developmentally appropriate discussions and ongoing dialogue, children will grow to understand the necessity of the medications and will be allowed to develop a sense of independence regarding their bodies and health.

Adolescence. Teenage development brings with it its own complications. As adolescents struggle to achieve independence, some find medication adherence, or the lack thereof, an obvious way to assert their autonomy. Adolescents may misperceive that they can be in control by making a choice as to whether or not to take their daily pills, as opposed to recognizing that by not taking their pills they may be giving control to the illness.

> *A teen whose parent was particularly overprotective–as a result of her guilt regarding HIV transmission–would gleefully talk in therapy about her one-upping her mother by not taking the pills.*

Teens often feel infallible and assume that they will persevere regardless of what medications they do or don't take. The long, often asymptomatic state of HIV infection provides little incentive to the adolescent to adhere to treatment (Smith Rogers et al., 2001). Unlike other chronic illnesses which may have a built-in positive and negative reinforcement system for levels of adherence, HIV treatment cause and effect can confuse any patient, let alone a teenager (ibid). The strong desire to be "normal" like everybody else, heightened in adolescence, is constantly challenged by HIV. Even routine medical appointments bring into consciousness an unwanted reminder of an undesired illness.

> *Teens talk openly about the burnout they feel with the medications and treatment. Frequent are the comments such as "I'm fine–why does everyone keep bothering me?" "I have never been sick–what is everyone so worried about? What's the point of taking these nasty pills?"*

The typical adolescent's focus on the 'here and now' complicates HIV treatment. The chronic, long-term nature of HIV treatment is a difficult concept for teenagers to comprehend and cope with. Therefore, strategies to assist with adherence must place special emphasis on unique ways to engage teenagers and maintain their care (Dodds et al., 2003).

Another significant issue that impedes the ability of children of all ages to adhere is the fact that there is no cure for HIV. How does one convince a child or teenager of the necessity of adherence when no matter how adherent they are, they will never be free of the disease? Studies have shown that adherence decreases with the length of time on treatment (Stone, 2001). In addition to the normal treatment fatigue and loss of motivation that comes with having to take long-term medications, there is the confounding decrease in hopefulness that many patients with HIV experience as they recognize that adherence will never lead to perfect health.

> *A teen said, "What is the point of all of this? Why should I suffer now with all these pills when I'm only going to end up dying like my mom?"*

Teenagers with HIV are also confronting the appropriate issues of their developmental stage such as dating, sexual experimentation, acting out, separation from parents/caregivers and increasingly strong peer relationships and influence. All these age appropriate challenges are complicated by the disease's inherent stigma and stress (Ledlie, 2001). The question of whether or not to disclose one's HIV status to sexual partners and friends may not only place an emotional burden on the teen, but also influences adherence directly and indirectly, consciously and unconsciously. In situations where the teen has chosen not to disclose, taking medications in front of peers or partners is not a viable option.

> *Even with new pharmaceutical methods of packaging and "un-HIV specific" gadgets for reminding them, teens complain that "it's obvious" if watches beep or beepers buzz and they have to take out their "vitamin pack" in front of peers. "People see these medications on the ads in the subway. There's no way to hide HIV from my friends, if I am seen with the pills."*

The complexity of the psychosocial context in which HIV+ children live seems to increase as children get older. In addition to complicated "teenage" issues, adolescents with HIV may have family concerns that confound their own medical and psychological needs.

We learn from studies of other chronic illnesses that the quality of family relationships impacts adherence (DeLambo et al., 2004). As important as family support may be for adherence, it follows that the interpersonal conflict within these relationships may have a destabilizing effect and negatively impact adherence (Wood et al., 2004). The typically ambivalent relationship that exists in the best of circumstances between parent and child during adolescence, can only complicate the adherence process. At times, teenagers act out as a way of asserting their independence. When a child who is HIV+ acts out, certain behaviors can be life threatening, such as avoidance of medical treatment, sexual activity and drug use.

Teenagers may live in unstable home environments, living between the homes of different family members and friends, many of whom have their own complicated problems. In the mind of the teen, these issues far outweigh her concerns regarding HIV. These factors of instability in the teen's life have proven to be some of the strongest correlates to adherence with the medical regimen (Martinez et al., 2000).

> *When a teenager has come to clinic after a fight with a parent and has been kicked out of the house, food, shelter, school, and maintaining relationships with those in his neighborhood are the issues that predominate.*

HIV families are often faced with issues of fragmented care; all family members are unlikely to attend the same medical clinic. In the rare clinics that provide services to both children and adults with HIV, often the HIV-negative family members need to attend a separate clinic.

> *One family talked about the burden of their appointment calendar–each day after school was filled with appointments throughout the city scheduled to address the financial, psychological, social, medical and concrete services that they needed to survive and thrive. The physical toll taken by "running around" (throughout 4 of the 5 boroughs of NYC) set the family up to fail.*

Parents and Caregivers' Experience of HIV

Pediatric adherence cannot be examined without exploring the caregiver's experience of HIV. Children are dependent on their caregivers; adherence to a medication regimen is but one of the many things for which HIV positive children must rely on others. However, there are multiple factors that impact a parent and caregiver's perception of the medications and treatment regimen.

Parents' illness as a factor in the adherence process. Parents may not have accepted their own HIV status, let alone that of their child. Administering medication to one's child forces an adult to confront his or her own health issues and the reality of the child's illness, which an HIV infected parent may not be prepared, or able, to do. One of the most frequently self-reported barriers to adherence is that medication is a reminder of one's HIV status (Ferguson et al., 2002). It may be easier for a parent to resist giving the child's medication, thus supporting the denial of his or her own illness.

When a child is diagnosed with HIV, regardless of the coping mechanisms of the parent, the child's medical condition requires immediate attention. The pediatric team asks parents and caregivers to assume responsibility for their children's adherence. Without assessing the emotional subtext of a parent's experience with medications, the potential for adherence failure is great. It is logical that an adult who has not been adherent himself, may not be adherent with the child's medication regimen. This is not true in all situations. There are some parents who are not able to take care of themselves but are able to do so for their children. Yet without a detailed assessment of the parent's relationship to adherence, an appropriate treatment plan cannot be formulated.

A parent who may be in the end-stage of her disease may not be physically able to take care of her child. Recognizing that you have reached a stage where you are unable to take care of your child is emotionally challenging, both in the relinquishing of responsibility, and in the outward acknowledgement of the severity of your own condition. It imposes perhaps two of life's most difficult issues to resolve: coming to terms with your own mortality and the welfare of your child.

Reactions to Medications. It is not unusual to experience side effects with the initiation of treatment: nausea, headaches, rashes or other symptoms (Williams, 1999). Parents may have had unpleasant side effects from the medication, and want to protect their child from a similar experience. When the outward functioning of a child appears good, there is little incentive to give medications with potential adverse effects. Being invisible, the benefits may seem only theoretical. There may also be the perception that while no harm is immediately apparent, there may be long-ranging consequences, still unstudied, which could emerge later in the child's life.

Caregivers often question the true efficacy of the medications. At the beginning of the epidemic they were told by their providers, that medications would help but only if their child were totally adherent. Many caregivers found that their children have survived and seem to be thriving despite sporadic adherence. This has further weakened the impetus to change to more adherent behavior.

Parents and caregivers often have misinformation about medications. In an era with easy Internet access, most people can go on-line and find information to support alternate theory of HIV or opinions of antiretroviral medication. It can be difficult to discern truth from fiction. Parents and caregivers do not always bring the information they learn online, or on the street, back to their health care providers for verification.

Other factors influencing adherence. Research in pediatric chronic illness has shown adherence to be correlated with caregivers' understandings of a regimen and its complexity (Thompson and Gustavson, 1996). There may be misunderstanding regarding the purpose and course of treatment. Viral loads and T-cell counts, the means of assessing the therapeutic value of the medications, are often unintelligible to parents and children. The enduring nature of HIV, coupled with the need for life-long medications, challenges everyday coping, future-oriented planning and goal setting. Dealing with a disease forever is daunting, even to high-functioning families with tremendous levels of support.

Minority patients have a long history of being the subjects of unethical medical research, leading to a lack of trust in the medical establishment (Savit, 1982; Pence, 1995). Patients often cite what they perceive to be the experimental nature of HIV treatment as a barrier to using HAART therapy (Ricther et al., 1995).

Other parents' guilt and sense of responsibility regarding the transmission of the disease makes confronting the child with anything unpleasant an impossible task.

> *A father of a teenage girl talked insightfully about his parenting;*
> *"I felt so badly that my beautiful baby had to go through this (HIV)*
> *that I never wanted to hurt her again. I let her have anything she*

wanted. Now that she's a teenager, I'm paying the price. Anytime I try to set a limit, she laughs."

"Chronic sorrow" may be a pervasive emotion for parents of a child with HIV as they cope with the knowledge that HIV is a life-long disease (Antle et al., 2001). The ultimately fatal nature of HIV has been shown to place a heavy emotional burden on parents of children with HIV, regardless of the child's health status (Weiner et al., 1995).

Drug use, depression and other mental health issues represent significant factors for HIV infected adults (Brackis-Cott, 2003). These problems may render parents incapable of addressing their children's health needs.

It felt so good to be high. I didn't have to think about all the bad things I'd done in my life, including hurting (my daughter). It was the only time I didn't feel like killing myself.

Whether or not drug use is a preexisting condition before the diagnosis, a parent may turn to substance abuse as a means of eradicating the co-morbid depression that often accompanies HIV. While temporarily giving the parent an escape, it also damages family functioning and makes it unlikely that HIV-related care will be obtained.

Children are severely impacted by a parent's death. When a parent dies of the same disease a child has, the impact is even greater. The implications for adherence are significant, both during the medical crises, and for the family in the period of adjustment long after the parent dies. The impact of the emotional legacy left behind when one parent dies of AIDS cannot be underscored.

As the child's mother lay dying of AIDS in the ICU, the child kept crying, "I'm going to die, I'm going to die." Watching her mother established a presentiment of her own future.

Cognitive and psychological factors for parents, in conjunction with those attributes of the child, highlight the complexity of achieving routine adherence. Without a full assessment of these and of all other psychosocial factors that impede access to care (transportation, financial issues, housing, domestic violence) providers cannot gauge how a family will respond to complicated medical regimens. Without a positive patient-provider relationship, the unfolding of the patient's life story may never occur.

Strategies for Improving Adherence

The challenges for adherence can be daunting, yet children are quick to come up with answers to what would make the medicines easier to take such as *"Make them taste better," "make the pills smaller,"* and *"make them once a week."* Unfortunately, these suggestions entail the assistance of drug companies. In the absence of grander societal solutions, given the opportunity, children generate rituals on their own to make the medications more palatable. *"Eating ice cream to kill the taste," "taking 3 sips of Ensure then rinsing with water," "sucking on a red candy before and after,"* are techniques children have created, empowering themselves, and improving adherence. Giving the child some authority regarding how the medicines are taken can improve adherence.

Adult patients' beliefs that they can make HIV medications fit into their lives have been shown to be predictive of good adherence (Cheever et al., 1999). It follows that by allowing children the opportunity to participate in their treatment and to plan adherence strategies, their sense of competency and belief in the feasibility of treatment will be heightened, thus improving adherence.

The reverse has also been highlighted: caregivers' perceptions that adherence is too difficult directly affects their ability to assist their children with complicated medical regimens (Reddington et al., 2000). Utilizing personalized calendars for children to check off doses taken is a technique that serves as a reminder, an acknowledgment of having taken the medication, and a way to partialize the overwhelming aspects of long-term adherence. Another way to empower children is to provide them with simplified, individualized education packets including photos of the medications. This activity gives children the tools and language to talk with providers fluently and expertly about their experiences. It also allows them information to share with family, friends and others in their social system, should they choose to disclose their HIV status.

There are resources to assist children in learning how to swallow pills (e.g., *www.acor.org*; *www.bayloraids.org*). Swallowing pills, versus drinking liquids, can simplify the process of taking medication. Educating and empowering the parent to teach the child this new skill has proven invaluable; both the child and the parent gain a new sense of mastery and often find the process (which usually involves candy and game-like strategies) a way of fostering positive familial interaction.

Families are encouraged to use other creative, concrete tools such as colorfully decorated pillboxes. Parents can be assisted in creating reward systems for adherent days and weeks. As the benefits of the medications are often cerebral rather than tangible, actual rewards concretize the process for children.

Often having an external monitoring agent is helpful in increasing adherence. Using a resource such as a visiting nurse or a pharmacy adherence program that routinely check administered doses, helps encourage the family to regularly adhere. Utilizing a resource that sees the family in the context of their home may lessen some of the anxiety that can inhibit communication at the clinic visits.

Psychosocial group work fostering interaction with others handling similar situations can be helpful to both children and caregivers. The mutual support received by knowing that others are coping and feeling successful with the same challenges can be motivating and supportive (Richter et al., 1998). Pairing children with others on the same regimen and providing opportunities for them to share their experiences, whether in the clinic setting or in the community, allows them to brainstorm on coping strategies, "compare notes," and offer each other support. Many HIV+ children ruminate privately about the consequences of HIV, but show few outward signs of distress (Bose et al., 1994). Creating a safe environment to elicit discussion encourages children to share their internal experiences.

Increasing psychosocial programming for both children and families can be beneficial. Many families are not only isolated by the secrecy surrounding HIV, but may also be away from their home countries, where they cannot return due to immigration issues or lack of medical care. When the context of the extended family is missing, other resources can be implemented to support both the family and the treatment.

Open communication is the cornerstone for any approach to improve adherence. Asking both the parent and child directly about their perceptions of adherence has proven to be simple and reliable (Van Dyke, 2002). Not only is this an efficient method, it empowers the patient by putting both child and parent in the position of being the "expert."

An overlooked strategy for providers is to view adherence in the context of the multiple roles played by the child or adolescent: child, peer, student, sexual partner (Dodds et al., 2003). This approach allows the provider and patient to recognize the many factors that cause adherence to remain a fluid, not static, concept.

Providers have an obligation to learn about patients' culture, perceptions of health and past experience with treatment. By allowing family members the opportunity to educate providers about their experiences and perceptions of illness, treatment and HIV, a common ground for initiating and maintaining treatment will be established.

A family-focused care approach would ensure the greatest ease to the patient and the best chance at forming trusting partnerships between the family and the members of the health care community. Instead of the parallel illnesses complicating matters, family-focused care would streamline issues with medical providers. In addition, sites that addressed all aspects of care, including: care of the healthy family members and the multiple psychosocial factors that confront the family, would alleviate the potential burden families face as they try to make sense of their complex worlds.

Whatever method is chosen to improve adherence, it is the process of collaboratively creating a plan among providers, child and family that is beneficial. It is critical to view any measure taken to improve adherence through the subjective lens of the unfolding relationship between the medical team, the patient and family, and all the biopsychosocial factors that affect HIV infected families. While this can be overwhelming, without it, the vision of adherence is significantly hindered.

Hanging over the process of adherence for any HIV+ child, like the "sword of Damocles," is the potential or actual death of one or both parents, other family members or of the children themselves. This reality influences the child's perception of life, both in its possibilities and vulnerabilities.

The trauma children experience when any parent dies has been well documented (Christ, 2000). Children with HIV are no less vulnerable than other children whose parents have died. In addition, they may not have the same resources available to them to help them cope with loss. Compounding the already present stressors that HIV+ children face due to their own health, the multiple losses amplify the tremendous emotional burden.

The connection established with providers and the joint efforts made to improve adherence give HIV+ children and their families an avenue for discussion, support and hope. These relationships and efforts represent a concern for the future. The emotional bond that is formed, with its attention to health maintenance and the goal of optimal health, empowers children to be forward thinking and forward acting. Having a sense of the future enables children to be emotionally more engaged in the process of adherence.

REFERENCES

Antle, BJ, Wells, LM, Goldie, RS, DeMatteo, D and King, SM. (2002). Challenges of parenting for families living with HIV/AIDS. *Social Work*, 46(2), 159-169.

Bose, S, Moss, HA, Brouwers, P, Pizzo, P and Lorion, R. (1994). Psychological Adjustment of Immunodeficiency Virus-Infected School Age Children. *Developmental and Behavioral Pediatrics*, 15(3), S26-S33.

Brackis-Cott, E, Mellins, CA, Abrams, E, Reval, T. and Dolezel, C. (2003). Pediatric HIV Medication Adherence: The Views of Medical Providers from Two Primary Care Programs. *Journal of Pediatric Health Care*, 17(5), 252-260.

Bryne, M, Honig, J, Jugrau, A, Heffernan, SM and Donahue, MC. (2002). Achieving Adherence with Antiretroviral Medications for Pediatric HIV Disease. *The AIDS Reader*, 151-165.

Cheever, LW and Wu, AW. (1999). Medication Adherence Among HIV Infected Patients: Understanding the Complex Behavior of Taking This Complex Therapy. *Current Infectious Disease* 1(4), 401-407.

Christ, G. 2000. *Helping Children's Grief: Surviving a Parent's Death from Cancer*. New York: Oxford University Press.

Cincotta, N. (2004). The End of Life at the Beginning of Life: Working with Dying Children and Their Families. In *Living with Dying: A Handbook for End-of-Life Practitioners*, Edited by Joan Berzoff and Phyllis Silverman, Columbia University Press, NY.

Cincotta, N. (2003). The Journey of Middle Childhood: Who Are Latency Age Children? In *Developmental Theories Throughout the Life Cycle*. Edited by Sonia G. Austrian. Columbia University Press NY.

Cincotta, N. (1993). Psychosocial Issues in the World of Children with Cancer. *Cancer*, 71, S3251-3260.

Delambo, KE, Ievers-Landis, CE, Drotar, D and Quittner, AL. (2004) Association of Observed Family Relationship Quality and Problem-solving Skills with Treatment Adherence in Older Children and Adolescents with Cystic Fibrosis. *Journal of Pediatric Psychology*, 29(5), 343-353.

Dodds, S., Blakley, T, Lizzotte, JM, Friedman, LB, Shaw, K, Martinez, J., Siciliano, C, Walker, LE, Sotheran, JL, Sell, RL, Botwinick, G, Johnson, RL and Bell, D. (2003) Retention, Adherence, and Compliance: Special Needs of HIV-Infected Adolescent Girls and Young Women. *Journal of Adolescent Health*, 33(2), 39-45.

Ferguson, TF, Stewart, KE, Funkhouser, E, Tolson, J, Westfall, AO and Saag, MS. (2002). Patient-perceived Barriers to Antiretroviral Adherence: Associations with Race. *AIDS Care*, 14(5): 607-617.

Fogarty L, Roter D, Larson, S, Burke, J., Gillespie, J. and Levy R. (2002). Patient Adherence to HIV Medication Regimens: A Review of Published and Abstract Reports. *Patient Education and Counseling*, 46(2), 93-108.

Friedland GH and Williams, A. (1999). Attaining Higher Goals in HIV Treatment: The Central Importance of Adherence. *AIDS*, 13, S61-72.

Ginsburg, HP, Opper, S. 1998, Piaget's Theory of Intellectual Development. Englewood Cliffs, NJ; Apprentice Hall.

Goode, M, McMaugh, A, Crisp, J, Wales, S and Ziegler, JB (2003). Adherence Issues In Children and Adolescents Receiving Highly Active Antiretroviral Therapy. *AIDS Care,*. 15(3), 403-8.

Hutton, N. Management of Pediatric HIV Infection. 1998. Johns Hopkins University Division of Infectious Disease and AIDS Services. Conference II on HIV/AIDS, Brazil.

Ledlie, S. (2001) The Psychosocial Issues of Children with Perinatally Acquired HIV Disease Becoming Adolescents: A Growing Challenge for Providers. *AIDS Care*, 15(5), 231-236.

Martinez, J, Bell, D, Camacho, R, Henry-Reid, LM, Bell, M, Watson, C and Rodriguez, F. (2000). Adherence to Antiviral Drug Regimens in HIV-infected Adolescent Patients Engaged in Care in a Comprehensive Adolescent and Young Adult Clinic. *J Natl. Med Assoc*, 92(2), 55-61.

Murphy, DA, Sarr, M, Durako, SJ, Moscicki, A, Wilson, CM and Muenz, LR. (2003). Barriers to HAART Adherence Among Human Immunodeficiency Virus-Infected Adolescents. *Archives of Pediatric & Adolescent Medicine*, 157(3), 249-255.

Patterson, DL, Swindells, S, Mohr, J, Brester, M, Vergis, M, Squier et al. (2000). Adherence to Protease Inhibitor Therapy and Outcomes in Patients with HIV Infection. *Annals of Internal Medicine*, 1333, 21-30.

Pence, GE. Past Abuses of Human Research Subjects: The Tuskegee Study. (1995). In *Classic Cases in Medical Ethics*, 2nd Edition, McGraw-Hill.

Reddington C, Cohen J, Baldillo A, Toye M, Smith D, Kneut C, Demaria A, Bertolli J, and Hsu H. (2000). Adherence to Medication Regimens Among Children with Human Immunodeficiency Virus Infection. *Pediatric Infectious Disease Journal*, 19(12), 1148-1153.

Ricther, R, Michaels, M, Carlson, B and Coates, TJ. (19989). Motivators and Barriers to Use of Combination Therapies in Patients with HIV Disease. CAPS Monograph.

Savitt, TL. The Use of Blacks for Medical Experimentation and Demonstration in the Old South. (1982). *The Journal of Southern History*. XLVIII(3), 331-348.

Sherman, BF, Bonanno, GA, Weiner, LS and Battles, HB. (2000) When Children Tell their Friends they Have HIV: Possible Consequences for Psychological Well-being and Disease Progression. *Psychosomatic Medicine*, 62, 238-247.

Smith, RA, Miller, S, Murphy, DA, Tanney, M and Fortune, T. (2001). The TREAT (therapeutic regimens enhancing adherence in teens) Program: Theory and Preliminary Results. *Journal of Adolescent Health*, 29(3), 30-38.

Speece, MW, Brent, SB. Children's Understanding of Death: A Review of Three Components of a Death Concept. (1984). *Child Development*, 55(5), 1671-1678.

Steele, RG and Grauer, D. (2003). Adherence to Antiretroviral Therapy for Pediatric HIV Infection: Review of the Literature and Recommendations for Research. *Clinical Child and Family Psychology Review*, 2003, 6(1), 17-30.

Stone, VE. (2001). Strategies for Optimizing Adherence to Highly Active Antiretroviral Therapy: Lessons from Research and Clinical Practice. *Clinical Infectious Diseases*, 33, 865-872.

Thompson, RJ, Gustavson, KE. (1996). Adaptation to Chronic Childhood Illnesses. Washington DC: American Psychological Association. 1996.

Van Dyke, RB, Lee, S, Johnson, GM, Wiznia, A, Mohan, K, Stanley, K et al. (2002). Reported Adherence as a Determinant of Response to Highly Active Antiretroviral Therapy in Children Who Have Human Immunodeficiency Virus Infection. *Pediatrics*, 109(4), 61-68.

Watson, DC, Collins-Jones, TL and Lovelace, S. (1999). Antiretroviral Therapy of Pediatric HIV Infection: Making Hope a Reality. *AIDS Patient Care and STDs*, 13(10), 587-599.

Weiner, L, Moss, H, Davidson, R, Fair, C. Pediatrics: The Emerging Psychosocial Challenges of the AIDS Epidemic. (1992). *Child and Adolescent Social Work Journal*, 9(5), 381-407.

Weiner L, Fair, C, Pizzo, P. (1993). Care for the Child with HIV Infection and AIDS. In: Armstrong-Dailey A, Goltzer SZ, editors. *Hospice Care for Children*. New York: Oxford University Press.

Weiner L, Riekert, KA, Theut, S, Steinberg, SM and Pizzo, P (1995). Parental Psychological Adaptation and Children with HIV: A Follow-Up Study. *AIDS Patient Care*, 9:233-239.

Williams AB. (1999). New Horizons: Antiretroviral Therapy in 1997. *Journal of the Association of Nurses in AIDS Care*, 8, 26-38.

Wood SA; Tobias, C; McCree, J. (2004). Medication Adherence for HIV Positive Women Caring for Their Children: In Their Own Words. *AIDS CARE*, 16(7), 909-913.

Patient-Provider Relationships, HIV, and Adherence: Requisites for a Partnership

Arlyn Apollo, MD, MPH
Sarit A. Golub, PhD
Milton L. Wainberg, MD
Debbie Indyk, PhD

SUMMARY. This paper analyzes data collected through focus groups of patients at an outpatient AIDS clinic at a New York medical center. Seven focus groups were conducted with 42 HIV+ patients, and verbatim transcripts of focus group sessions were analyzed through a combination of ethnographic and content analysis. We examined patients' reports of interactions with and attitudes toward their providers and attempted to define what elements in the provider-patient relationship are necessary to enable patients to become more integrally involved in the management of their illness. Participants' statements emerged as consistent with three themes: (a) dynamics of provider-to-patient communication; (b) dynamics of patient-to-provider communication; and (c) dynamics of collabora-

---

Arlyn Apollo, MD, MPH, is affiliated with New York Presbyterian Hospital, New York, NY. Sarit A. Golub, PhD, is affiliated with Queens College, City University of New York. Milton L. Wainberg, MD, is affiliated with the New York Psychiatric Institute, Columbia University. Debbie Indyk, PhD, is affiliated with the Mount Sinai School of Medicine, New York, NY.

[Haworth co-indexing entry note]: "Patient-Provider Relationships, HIV, and Adherence: Requisites for a Partnership." Apollo, Arlyn et al. Co-published simultaneously in *Social Work in Health Care* (The Haworth Press, Inc.) Vol. 42, No. 3/4, 2006, pp. 209-224; and: *The Geometry of Care: Linking Resources, Research, and Community to Reduce Degrees of Separation Between HIV Treatment and Prevention* (ed: Debbie Indyk) The Haworth Press, Inc., 2006, pp. 209-224. Single or multiple copies of this article are available for a fee from The Haworth Document Delivery Service [1-800-HAWORTH, 9:00 a.m. - 5:00 p.m. (EST). E-mail address: docdelivery@haworthpress.com].

209

tion. Each of these themes is discussed in terms of its implications for creating patient-provider relationships based on mutual-participation, and requisites for effecting meaningful patient-provider partnerships are outlined. *[Article copies available for a fee from The Haworth Document Delivery Service: 1-800-HAWORTH. E-mail address: <docdelivery@haworthpress.com> Website: <http://www.HaworthPress.com> © 2006 by The Haworth Press, Inc. All rights reserved.]*

KEYWORDS. Communication, collaboration, patient-provider

It is easier to prescribe than to come to an understanding of the patient.

–*Franz Kafka, The Country Doctor*

In a 1956 discussion on the philosophy of medicine, Szasz and Hollender described three models of the physician-patient relationship: activity-passivity, guidance cooperation, and mutual participation. The first model, activity-passivity, depicts a situation in which the patient neither questions nor contributes at all to treatment. The second model, guidance-cooperation–was, for many years, considered the standard traditional model for clinical practice (Wirtz, Cribb, & Barber, 2005). The patient presents to a provider and describes his or her symptoms. The provider decides upon a treatment plan and expects the patient to follow it. The patient assumes that the provider has some special knowledge that he or she does not have, thereby creating a paternalistic relationship with a significant power differential between the two players.

The third paradigm is mutual participation, in which the two participants have approximately equal power and are mutually interdependent. Treatment programs are offered by the provider, but are discussed and implemented in consultation with the patient. When these three models were first proposed (almost 50 years ago), physician-patient relationships based on mutual participation were virtually non-existent (Szasz & Hollender, 1956). Since that time, both physicians and other care providers have embraced models of mutual participation (Roter & Hall, 1992; Henbest & Stewart, 1989; Wirtz et al., 2005). Research suggests that increasing patients' sense of self-efficacy can improve self-management of chronic illness (Kern, Penick, & Hamby, 1996), and increasing assertiveness and active participation in treatment improves clinical symptoms (Kaplan, Greenfield, & Ware, 1989).

However, even in the context of a mutual-participation model of care, the challenges associated with treating individuals living with chronic illness require an almost constant renegotiation and redefinition of patient-provider relationships. In Szasz and Hollender's original model, mutual participation is "characterized by a high degree of empathy, has elements often associated with the notions of friendship and partnership and the imparting of expert advice . . . The search for [what is best for the patient] becomes the essence of the therapeutic interaction. The patient's own experiences furnish indispensable information for eventual agreement as to what 'health' might be for him" (Szasz & Hollender, 1956, p. 168). This articulation recognizes the extent to which a model of mutual participation is a "moving target," which must be tailored to the experiences of each patient. Mutual participation is at the heart of patient-level approaches to the new geometry of care (Rier & Indyk, this volume), in which patients' experiences are considered important sources of information and continuing education for the providers who treat them.

But a commitment to a mutual-participation model is much easier said than done. Providing this type of care–rooted in empathy, partnership, flexibility–is extraordinarily difficult to negotiate. This article examines data collected through focus groups with patients at a designated AIDS Center and attempts to frame key issues that inform the development of a successful mutual-participation relationship between patient and provider.

METHOD

Participants

Participants were forty-two HIV-positive patients (24 males and 18 females) of Mount Sinai Medical Center's Jack Martin Fund Clinic (JMFC), a designated AIDS Center in East Harlem, New York City. Participants ranged in age from 25 to 61, with a mean and median of 40. Twenty participants (49%) self-identified as Latino(a) and seventeen (41%) identified as African American. The majority of the sample (66%) had only high-school level education; three participants (7%) had a college degree. Thirty-five participants (87.5%) reported having taken protease inhibitors; of these, two reported starting protease inhibitors and two reported stopping protease inhibitors in the last month.

Design and Procedure

Participants attended one of seven focus groups, which ranged in size from four to eight participants each. All patients of the JMFC were eligible for participation. Study participants were recruited in the clinic waiting room using both active and passive recruitment techniques (Morgan, 1990). Focus group questions were developed by a multidisciplinary team of HIV providers (an infectious disease specialist, a psychiatrist, a social worker, and a behavioral scientist), and focus groups were conducted using semi-structured questionnaires. Each focus group session lasted approximately two hours. Participants were given a $15 Metrocard (transportation voucher) in appreciation of their participation. Focus group sessions were audio-taped.

Data Analysis

Verbatim transcripts of the audio-taped focus group sessions were analyzed through a combination of ethnographic and content analysis. While these two methods are often described separately, their combination–the utilization of both systematic tallying and close readings of direct quotations–is believed to enhance the strength of interpretation (Morgan, 1990; Ely, 1993). One goal of this study was to identify determinants of patient non-adherence to medication regimens; these findings are discussed elsewhere (Golub et al., this volume). In this article, we focus specifically on findings that inform aspects of productive patient-provider relationships. Below, results are presented in an integrative fashion designed to highlight key findings and suggest important areas for further systematic inquiry.

RESULTS

Overall, participant responses could be coded into three categories, each vital to the negotiation of a relationship of mutual participation: (a) dynamics of provider-to-patient communication; (b) dynamics of patient-to-provider communication; and (c) dynamics of collaboration between patient and provider. Each of these three categories is explained below, and is discussed in terms of its implications for improving a model of mutual participation between patient and provider.

Dynamics of Provider-to-Patient Communication: Lost in Translation

Communicating what is most important. Providers are responsible for conveying a tremendous amount of information to a patient in any clinical encounter. For a model of mutual participation to be successful, providers are faced with the task of communicating not only what a patient needs to do to keep herself healthy, but also why these behaviors are so important to initiate and maintain. For HIV, the information providers hope to help patients truly understand include: the mechanics of combination therapy, the development of drug resistance, the importance of maintaining strict adherence to medication schedules, as well as a host of other self-management and health promotion behaviors (dietary guidelines, reducing substance use, safer sex practices, etc.). In a rush to provide information, providers may assume that their message has been sent, but may not accurately assess the degree to which it has been misunderstood in interpretation. The patient does not raise issues regarding the misinterpretation, because he is not aware of it himself. For example, Christina (all names are pseudonyms) reported that she would often forget her evening dose of medication, but did not understand the potential consequences of this non-adherence:

> I was surprised because I thought I knew what I was really doing. I was totally off and it shocked me in a way because I thought he was going to say, "good, at least you still taking them," but he did not say that . . . I was really shocked today when he said that to me because I thought long as the pills was still in my system that I was OK.

Several patients also believed that it was acceptable to miss doses periodically, for example, while on vacation. An even more striking example of miscommunication between provider and patient was reported by another participant:

> Antonio: I want to take a couple of drinks and all that . . . and to forget . . . so that day I don't take the medication at all . . .
>
> Interviewer: The doctor told you it's not good to drink [while taking the pills]?

Antonio: Yeah, he said that I wasn't supposed to drink while I was on medication.

Antonio thought that he was following his doctor's advice: combining alcohol and his HIV medications could be harmful, so on days that Antonio wanted to drink, he simply stopped taking his HIV medication. Each member of the dyad in this situation thought that he understood what the other was saying, but the relative importance of the provider's two statements–taking medication is important; don't combine alcohol and the medications–was lost in translation. Most likely, Antonio's provider assumed that telling him that alcohol and his medications didn't mix would prevent him from drinking; Antonio perceived the message as advice about how to integrate drinking into his treatment regimen. Communicating what is most important also requires providers to think through the trade-offs that patients must make every day in managing their illness, and imagine how these choices might play out. Enhancing mutual-participation may mean providing information that can inform priority-setting for patients, identifying the medical (and psychological) consequences of different courses of action.

Dealing with side effects. Another critical aspect of provider-to-patient communication that emerged out of the focus group data was the importance of assisting patients in anticipating and making sense of the side-effects of their medication. Even the newest drug treatment regimens can induce side effects ranging from unpleasant to intolerable, and patients look to their providers to help them decide how much they are able–or willing–to bear. Several participants expressed extreme dissatisfaction with not being warned about the possibility of neurological side effects to their medications:

I didn't know where you get [neuropathy] . . . I didn't know what it was . . . the doctor didn't tell me . . .–Eva

. . . I just said well let me try this, not knowing . . . just knowing basic things that it could cause, but she never got into detail–my doctor–about what the side effects are. . . . they don't mention anything about it affecting your brain in any sort of way.–Gloria

In contrast, according to some patients, knowing what to expect may alleviate some fears about the medications. It may help to know that certain side effects can be considered normal reactions to treatment, and may, in some cases, abate over time. Discussions of side effects in the clinical encounter represent another responsibility of providers, in which they provide both textbook knowledge and expertise derived from experience with many other patients. In David's case, access to a nurse and their discussion of side effects supported his adherence:

> When I first experienced the side effects from nausea, I called up the nurse immediately and told her about it and she got back to me and told me that it was a side effect and that it would last awhile or maybe a couple of weeks and that kept me, that is actually what kept me going . . . knowing that I only had to put up with this for a little while made it much easier just to continue taking the medicine.

A gesture is worth a thousand words. Another theme that was articulated by multiple participants was a frustration with their providers for speaking in a manner the participants found too complicated or confusing. As David put it:

> Me, I'm the type of patient like when I go in and sit down with the doctor, he be talking a language that I don't think, you know, very many people can speak. So I'm just sitting there waiting till they get to English and they tell me take this two times a day, and I say, OK thank you and I go home and do that.

A provider's failure to translate technical language into terms the patient can understand may be a critical source of misunderstanding. Furthermore, technical language can create a barrier between provider and patient, and may prevent patients from feeling as though they can relate. It may also magnify existing perceived socio-cultural barriers. Compounding misunderstandings related to language barriers, many participants also explained that their providers' *nonverbal* communication left them feeling alienated. Nonverbal communication may be a key contributor to the relationship between patients and providers, as it conveys information about affect and attitude through touch, facial and body movements, and tone of voice. It may be more revealing than the spoken word; construction of sentences requires conscious effort and control, whereas nonverbal messages often escape control and may be more difficult to withhold. Unspoken communication is believed to be the principal medium for expressing information about emotions and attitudes and is thought to override verbal information when there is a conflict in the two channels. In some situations, patients place more weight on the physician's nonverbal behavior than on spoken language (Blanck, Buck, & Rosenthal, 1986).

The following statement by Jane illustrates how volumes of information may be transmitted through a tactile gesture or lack thereof. This comprises several dimensions of separation as described above, including, most importantly, a lack of understanding:

> A doctor that walks in and greets me with his hand in his pockets saying "good afternoon, Miss X, I'm Dr. So-and-so." I don't want to talk to him. I want a doctor that's going to walk in with his hand out to say "Miss X, I'm Dr. So-and-so" and make first contact, because if your hands are in your pocket you're for money, and say what would you do if you were in my shoes? You can never figure that out because you'll never be there . . . you see this is what I'm saying . . . these doctors are listening but they're not listening.

Studies have shown that physicians who scored higher on tests of nonverbal communication skill were associated with a higher level of patient satisfaction (DiMatteo, Hays & Prince, 1986). In these studies, a forward lean, eye contact, and maintaining close distance prevailed over verbal behavior in communicating empathy. A lack of eye contact may be perceived as a lack of compassion. Toni acted out a typical scenario with her physician:

> Sometimes they do, they just push you off, "how you feeling, Toni?" [miming, writing on a pad, not looking up]. "Well you know doctor I have some pain . . . " [Still not looking up] "OK well we'll make an appointment for you in 6 weeks . . ."

> Interviewer: Is it lack of eye contact?

> Toni: Just lack of everything . . . they don't . . . when you walk in, it's like they don't see you . . . you're just a piece of paper that they write . . .

> The combination of these two elements of communication–speaking in "plain English" and communicating attention through non-verbal behavior–are critical components of any mutual-participation relationship. The foundation of Szasz and Hollender's model (1956) is, as mentioned above, empathy, partnership, and

friendship. Each of these features is possible only if providers are truly "talking" to patients, both verbally and non-verbally.

Dynamics of Patient-to-Provider Communication: Are You Listening?

A mutual-participation model of patient-provider interaction is consistent with an approach that recognizes HIV-infected individuals as the new "locus of control" over HIV treatment and prevention (Indyk & Golub, this volume). For HIV management to be successful, not only must HIV-positive patients commit to following their medication regimens, they must also integrate HIV management into almost every aspect of their lives. For this reason, it is critical for providers to listen to patients, assess their readiness for initiating (and maintaining) treatment, and consider the competing concerns that affect their lives.

Readiness for treatment. The mutual participation model acknowledges that a patient may not be ready to begin treatment. It is believed that the likelihood of success in maintaining a treatment regimen is enhanced when both participants determine the regimen based on information about patient readiness. Patients need to be able to voice their own individual barriers to self-management; maintenance of treatment is more likely if the patient demonstrates a certain level of readiness to begin.

Beginning the right treatment at the right time is a key strategy in promoting self-management. One recommendation for further research is the creation of a tool to be used by providers in order to determine patient readiness to begin treatment, and to identify characteristics of a regimen that would be most suitable for a given patient's lifestyle. Likewise, a good rapport allows for both parties to participate in changing the regimen. Instead of stopping her regimen, Irene spoke with her doctor and agreed to switch from one combination of medications to another:

> He's a nice doctor so he agrees with it and then when I stopped the medication I told him before time that I wanted to stop the medication so he agrees with it and then we decided to change. We decided together which one would suit me better.

Teaching the provider. The second aspect of patient-to-provider communication identified by focus-group participants is the extent to which patients can provide information to their providers beyond a mere litany of symptoms. A model of mutual-participation requires shared decision-making, and demands that the patient often assume a teaching role. Focus group participants differed in the extent to which they took active roles in bringing information to their providers, but all participants acknowledged the extent to which patients possess unique knowledge about their illness:

> They're not God. They just read and they study these things. They go by what you're telling them. You have to help them with it. They don't know.–Steve

> They're looking at it from you know this textbook standpoint compared to looking at it from actual life. Cause what's in the textbook, I believe it always differs a little bit from what you are actually going through. Like when I tried to explain to my doctor about this . . . she told me I didn't need it. I know I need it . . . I know what my appetite is like, you don't know, all you know is what I tell you . . . maybe you get your conclusions from numbers, basically . . . but what is normal for [the patient]?–David

The importance of providers' learning from the unique experiences of their patients should not construed as a mandate to involve patients in every aspect of their treatment. Patients vary in how much help and attention they want and need to manage illness, and perhaps one of the most difficult tasks for a provider is determining the patient's level of comfort in sharing authority over his or her treatment. The chronic illness literature strongly suggests that patients should be offered a role in the decision-making process, but that patients may not choose to do so. Some research suggests that approximately two-thirds of cancer patients felt that the doctor should be the primary decision-maker (Sutherland, Llewellyn-Thomas, Lockwood, Tritchler, & Till, 1989); other research has shown that nearly one-third of cancer patients preferred not to participate at all in treatment-related decisions (Blanchard, Labrecque, Ruckdeschel, & Blanchard, 1988).

Some patients may not be ready to enter a partnership at the onset of treatment, and may become increasingly comfortable in that role if they are encouraged to do so. Because managing life with HIV is a full-time occupation, there is a greater onus on patients to be effective communicators, and on providers to provide ample opportunity for the transfer of information. As advocated in models of the new geometry of care for

HIV (Rier & Indyk, this volume), information transfer from patient to provider is critical to successful management and support.

Dynamics of Collaboration: Attention to the Experience of Illness

The final dynamic vital to the negotiation of a relationship of mutual participation relates to the collaboration between patients and providers in the management of HIV as a chronic illness. Beyond clear communication in the context of the clinical encounter, a model of mutual participation requires recognition of the patient's experience of illness, and the ways in which providers can support and ease its burden. Dynamics of patients' experience of illness as they relate specifically to determinants of treatment adherence are discussed elsewhere (Golub et al., this volume). Below, we discuss issues raised by patients regarding the experience of illness as it relates to fostering productive patient-provider relationships.

"I have to live that life." Not surprisingly, many patients reported difficulty in patient-provider communication that they attributed to an inability of their provider to truly understand their experience of living with HIV:

> I don't care what they got to say because they're not taking the medication . . . I'm taking it . . . I'm feeling what's going on with the medication, so you can't tell me this is happening when I'm telling you something else is happening because I'm feeling this. . . . you're not in my skin . . . just because your [other] patients don't have that reaction doesn't mean I'm not having this reaction . . . –Cassandra

> You're looking at that doctor and saying, 'This doctor don't understand nothing I'm going through.' First of all we're people of color . . . so you don't understand that . . . you don't know what it is to be an addict because you never shot no drugs . . . you don't know how our self-esteem is . . . you don't know what level it's on.–Toni

The quotations above illustrate two fundamental challenges to creating genuine mutual-participation relationships. The first are dynamics of difference–most notably those of race and class–that often exist between patient and provider. Issues of race and class are not always present, of course, but when they are, they can often seem too imposing to adequately address or overcome. The second challenge raised by these quotations is the extent to which an HIV diagnosis exists within an individual's life, a life that is almost always complex and filled with competing (and sometimes more pressing) demands. One approach to meeting this challenge is to draw on the resources of individuals and organizations with which the patient feels closer, or more able to connect. Linda explained the extent to which she felt that community-based organizations were an important resource to provide the care and support she needs:

> A white person out of college coming out of the book cannot tell me nothing about the street . . . you cannot help me. I need the CBO to help me because these people are from the ghetto just like I am. . . .

Other participants explained that peer educators, other individuals who are living with HIV, can make a difference in terms of both information and support: .

> The peer educator could–like I'm talking to you–we could begin to say "What are you taking? Did you try it like this? You know, I did it like this." Then there would be an understanding . . . because the doctors don't understand . . . they can't understand the stress she's going through at home.–Toni

Within this context, another strategy is to acknowledge difference, but to focus on the extent to which these differences are simply one part of the whole person the provider is trying to treat and support. Patients who felt the least distance from their providers were those who felt that their providers recognized and cared for them as "whole people." As Larry put it:

> [My doctor] not only cares about you that you're taking your medication, she cares about everything else . . . you know, how are things in your personal life, like how are things at home? How are things with your family . . . how are you feeling mentally as well as physically?

When providers are able to focus on the "whole person" they are trying to support, empathy and attention flow naturally, and patients feel more able to collaborate in their care.

Issues of access. The final two issues raised by focus group participants as they relate to the model of mutual participation are systemic in
nature. The promise of attending to a patient's "whole person" is inherently constrained by the logistics of a patient-provider encounter, which
usually lasts a maximum of twenty minutes and is often driven by the
completion of forms and other paperwork. The typical HIV patient sees
his or her physician once every four to six weeks, must convey all aspects of his or her health status, including experience with medications,
as well as receive feedback and information on health management, in a
20-minute encounter. As Cassandra stated:

> I have to live that life, and by me coming to see you once a month
> and I let you know what's going on . . . you have to really listen to
> what I have to say to you.

The dynamics of both communicating and listening have been discussed above, but this quotation also draws attention to the extent to
which patient-provider collaboration requires "presence," in the face of
competing demands for both patient and provider.

The second issue raised by patients relates the literal, physical meaning
of this presence–their ability to contact, speak with, or see their provider in
a timely fashion. Access to providers was cited by many participants as a
barrier to management of their illness and treatment. Paul explained that he
was experiencing side effects from his medication but was unable to make
an appointment with his physician. After trying for a week, he reported:

> I just stopped [taking the pills] so I don't have to worry about that
> [the side effects]. I just take my own chances on it . . . I'm not
> gonna take no more of this medicine, and you know you're not get-
> ting the primary care you're supposed to get taking it, you know.

The demands of mutual participation and true collaboration between
provider and patient require a difficult commitment to creating care systems that enable patients to access their providers.

CONCLUSION

Taken together, the issues raised by these patients draw attention to
critical components of mutual-participation relationships between patients and providers, and suggest several recommendations for guide-

lines for future practice. In terms of provider-to-patient communication, participants' statements highlight several key issues. First, it is critical for providers to "check-in" with patients after communicating complicated or emotionally charged information, to make sure the patient understands the information in the way the provider intends. Antonio's experience stopping his medication because he wanted a drink and his doctor told him that alcohol and his medication shouldn't mix is related to this point, but suggests another level of patient-provider understanding. Providers need to engage patients in conversations about the trade-offs inherent in HIV-management, in the hopes that patients and providers can come to a mutual understanding of priorities. Since infected individuals will be living with the virus for the rest of their lives, provider recommendations must give patients the tools to make choices that will enable them to live these lives fully. A discussion like this one might have helped Antonio identify harm-reduction type strategies when he wanted to have a drink.

Discussion of priorities is inextricably related to the third issue raised by patients, the importance of anticipating and preparing for upcoming changes, be they increased side effects or changes related to other aspects of living with HIV. The last two issues had to do with provider communication style: Participants stressed the importance of speaking in clear, non-technical language that they can easily understand, and the importance of non-verbal communication that suggest a genuine level of care.

In terms of patient-to-provider communication, the most important issue was the extent to which providers are open to listening and learning from their patients. Consistent with conceptions of horizontal knowledge transfer (Rier & Indyk, this volume), participants suggested that providers might learn information about HIV from their patients that is at least as valuable (if not more valuable) than the latest results of a clinical trial.

Participants' comments about patient-provider collaboration extended these sentiments, and focused on the extent to which mutual participation requires a recognition of patients' experience living with HIV day-to-day. Participants drew attention to the contradiction that they must often balance–HIV has the ability to overwhelm patients' lives even though the disease is only one small part of their everyday concerns. Participants stressed the extent to which their provider needed to treat their "whole person," which may also mean recruiting support from outside traditional care centers.

To return to our original definition of mutual participation, "the search for [what is best for the patient] becomes the essence of the therapeutic interaction" (Szasz & Hollender, 1959, p. 168). The requisites for a true partnership between patient and provider involve attention to the dynamics articulated above, and a commitment to care systems that support providers in making these types of communications possible.

REFERENCES

Blanchard, C.G., Labrecque, M.S., Ruckdeschel, J.C., & Blanchard, E.B. (1988). Information about decision-making preferences of hospitalized adult cancer patients. *Social Science and Medicine*, 27 (11), 1139-1145.

Blanck, P.D., Buck, R., & Rosenthal, R. (1986). *Nonverbal Communication in the Clinical Context*. University Park, PA: Pennsylvania State University Press.

DiMatteo, M.R., Hays, R.D., & Prince, L.M. (1986). Relationship of physicians' nonverbal communication skill to patient satisfaction, appointment noncompliance, and physician workload. *Health Psychology*, 5 (6), 581-594.

Ely, M. (1993) *Doing qualitative research: Circles within circles*. Bristol, PA: Falmer.

Golub, S.A., Indyk, D., & Wainberg, M.L. (this volume). Reframing HIV adherence as part of the experience of illness. *Social Work in Health Care*.

Henbest, R.J., & Stewart, M.A. (1989). Patient-centeredness in the consultation: A method for measurement. *Family Practice*. Vol. 6 (249).

Indyk, D., & Golub, S.A. (2005). The shifting locus of risk-reduction: The critical role of HIV infected individuals. *Social Work in Health Care*. 42(3/4), 113-132.

Kaplan, S.H., Greenfield, S., & Ware, J.E., Jr. (1989). Assessing the effect of physician-patient interactions on the outcomes of chronic disease. *Medical Care*, 27 (3 Suppl), S110-127.

Kern, R.M., Penick, J.M., & Hamby, R.D. (1996). Prediction of diabetic adherence using the BASIS-A inventory. *The Diabetes Educator*, 22 (4), 367-371.

Morgan, D.L. (1990). *Focus Groups as Qualitative Research*. Newbury Park, CA: Sage.

Rier, D.A., & Indyk, D. (2005). The rationale of interorganizational linkages to connect multiple sites of expertise, knowledge production, and knowledge transfer: An example from HIV/AIDS services for the inner city. *Social Work in Health Care* 42(3/4), 9-27.

Roter, D.L., & Hall, J.A. (1992). *Doctors Talking with Patients, Patients Talking with Doctors*. Westport, CT: Auburn House.

Sutherland, H.J., Llewellyn-Thomas, H.A., Lockwood, G.A., Tritchler, D.L., & Till, J.E. (1989). Cancer patients: Their desire for information and participation in treatment decisions. *Journal of Social Medicine*, 82 (5), 260-263.

Szasz, T.S. & Hollender, M.H. (1956). A contribution to the philosophy of medicine: The basic models of the doctor-patient relationship. *AMA Archives of Internal Med-*

icine, Reprinted in Stoeckle, J., (Ed.), Encounters between Patients and Doctors. Cambridge, MA: The MIT Press, 1987.

Wirtz, V., Cribb, A., & Barber, N. (2005). Patient-doctor decision-making about treatment within the consultation–a critical analysis of models. Social Science in Medicine, in press. Retrieved from the web, July 6, 2005. *doi:10.1016/j.socs cimed.2005.05.017*

HIV-Infected Individuals
as Partners in Prevention:
A Redefinition
of the Partner Notification Process

Sarit A. Golub, PhD

Debbie Indyk, PhD

SUMMARY. Over the past ten years, the advances that have turned HIV into a chronic illness have also highlighted the importance of integrating prevention and care in the fight against the epidemic. This integration involves not only the creation of new programs, but also a reexamination of the process through which services and supports are provided. In this article, HIV partner notification is used as a case example; the discussion includes: the shifting time frame within which partner notification occurs; the expanding role of HIV-positive individuals in effecting both disease management and prevention goals; the connection between partner-notification and behaviorally-based risk reduction; and the ethical implications of advances on the partner notification process. The authors argue that partner notification services must be located in the context of overall treatment for infected individuals, and demonstrate how a redefinition of the partner noti-

---

Sarit A. Golub, PhD, is affiliated with Queens College, City University of New York. Debbie Indyk, PhD, is affiliated with the Mount Sinai School of Medicine, New York, NY.

[Haworth co-indexing entry note]: "HIV-Infected Individuals as Partners in Prevention: A Redefinition of the Partner Notification Process." Golub, Sarit A., and Debbie Indyk. Co-published simultaneously in *Social Work in Health Care* (The Haworth Press, Inc.) Vol. 42, No. 3/4, 2006, pp. 225-235; and: *The Geometry of Care: Linking Resources, Research, and Community to Reduce Degrees of Separation Between HIV Treatment and Prevention* (ed: Debbie Indyk) The Haworth Press, Inc., 2006, pp. 225-235. Single or multiple copies of this article are available for a fee from The Haworth Document Delivery Service [1-800-HAWORTH, 9:00 a.m. - 5:00 p.m. (EST). E-mail address: docdelivery@haworthpress.com].

Available online at http://www.haworthpress.com/web/SWHC
doi:10.1300/J010v42n03_14

fication process can serve as a spring-board for ongoing prevention counseling and support. *[Article copies available for a fee from The Haworth Document Delivery Service: 1-800-HAWORTH. E-mail address: <docdelivery@haworth
press.com> Website: <http://www.HaworthPress.com> © 2006 by The Haworth
Press, Inc. All rights reserved.]*

KEYWORDS. Prevention, integration, treatment counseling

The term "partner notification" refers to a process by which individuals who may have been exposed to an infectious agent–e.g., HIV or
another sexually transmitted disease–are notified of their potential exposure. For many years, partner notification or "contact tracing" has
been used as an important public health tool to reduce the spread of
sexually transmitted infections (STIs). Individuals treated for STIs are
routinely asked to provide names and contact information for any recent sexual partners. These partners are then contacted by a public
health official and asked to come to a clinic for testing and treatment.
This type of contact tracing is anonymous; individuals are told of their
possible exposure, but the partner who named them as a contact is not
identified. In the STI model, patients receive test results, curative
treatment, and partner notification counseling in the same visit. No ongoing relationship with the patient is necessary, since the patient is no
longer infected.

In the early stages of the epidemic, HIV partner notification was
modeled after traditional STI contact tracing (Bayer & Toomey, 1992;
Ramstedt et al., 1990). Partner notification was placed within the context of HIV counseling and testing. Newly diagnosed individuals were
given a contact tracing interview, but partner notification remained
completely separate from any treatment or ongoing care plan.

THE SHIFT FROM PAST TO FUTURE PARTNERS

As mentioned above, contact tracing for STI infection focuses exclusively on *past* partners. The STI clinic can provide infected individuals
with curative treatment, so the index patient will not expose his or her
future partners to the STI. Before the advent of combination therapy,
partner notification for HIV infection was also focused almost exclusively on past partners. It was assumed that HIV-positive individuals

would have no future partners. This assumption was based both on the altruism of infected individuals in protecting the uninfected, and on the extent to which impending illness and death would make it impossible for infected individuals to continue sexual relationships.

Understanding HIV as a chronic illness shifts the time-frame within which partner notification efforts can and should occur. As HIV-positive individuals live longer and healthier lives, they will continue to have sexual or even needle sharing partners. And, unlike those infected with gonorrhea, chlamydia, or syphilis, HIV-positive individuals will continue to be infectious for the rest of their lives. Revised models of partner notification have acknowledged the importance of focusing on *current* partners; however, the shift in time frame must extend even further to include an infected individual's *future* partners. In addition to having partners with whom they are currently active and partners with whom they have been active in the past, HIV-positive individuals may have partners with whom they are considering becoming active in the future. These future partners can be considered "at imminent risk" and their notification is perhaps the most directly related to primary prevention goals.

But how does one identify–let alone notify–future partners? Placed within the frame of traditional partner notification processes, this idea is absurd: "Is there someone you have your eye on?" However, the acknowledgement of the importance of infected individuals' future partners highlights the extent to which the process of partner notification must move away from the point of testing or diagnosis and become part of the ongoing management of HIV. In this vein, partner notification must be seen as part of the process of disclosure and part of the process of risk-reduction. Each of these factors is discussed in detail below.

PARTNER NOTIFICATION REDEFINED:
A DISCLOSURE ASSISTANCE PROGRAM

Partner notification services for HIV infection have been extremely controversial. While many have argued that partner notification is a public health imperative, others have argued that mandating partner notification runs contrary to public health goals by discouraging infected individuals from seeking testing and treatment (Dimas & Richland, 1989). Guidelines released by the Centers for Disease Control and Prevention encourage partner counseling and referral services (PCRS), but do not mandate the specifics of PCRS programs (CDC, 1998). The majority of states have enacted legislation which requires medical professionals to report known partners of HIV-infected individuals (primarily spouses), but request–rather than require–reporting by HIV-positive patients themselves. However, this conception of partner notification still focuses on its importance for the lives of the contacts, while neglecting its power in the life of the HIV-positive individual.

Patient versus Provider Referral. There has been much debate over the relative merits of partner notification through patient referral, in which infected individuals self-disclose to their partners, versus partner notification through provider referral, in which partners names are given to a professional who notifies them without disclosing the identity of the index patient. Some studies have shown that provider referral is more effective in reaching past partners than is patient referral (Landis et al., 1992), and some have recommended focusing scarce resources on this method. However, expanding the time frame for partner notification also means expanding its goals. For past partners, the goal of partner notification remains contact tracing, which may be accomplished through either provider or patient referral. For current partners, the goal of partner notification moves beyond notification of past exposure to include prevention of future exposure as well. Anonymous provider referral for current partners (e.g., "*someone* with whom you are currently active is HIV-positive") does not fulfill prevention goals; if the notified individual has more than one partner she will not necessarily take precautions with the right one. As mentioned above, provider referral for future partners becomes almost ridiculous ("someone with whom you are *considering* becoming active is HIV-positive").

Therefore, the expanding time frame requires an expanding role for HIV-positive individuals and for the patient referral process. However, in order to be effective, patient referral and the process of self-disclosure must be supported more fully. More research must be conducted to determine which individuals may need extra help and what interventions and supports facilitate self-disclosure. While it is always a difficult process, disclosure may present an additional obstacle depending on external situations, individual resources and personal limitations.

While the stigma and discrimination associated with HIV-infection has clearly decreased since the early 1980s, HIV-positive individuals still face significant repercussions from disclosing their status. In a recent large-scale study of HIV-positive women, 44% reported negative consequences of disclosing their HIV-status, including loss of friends, being insulted or sworn at, and being rejected by their families (Gielen, Fogarty, O'Campo, Anderson, Keller, & Faden, 2000). HIV-infected women often have a history of being victims of violence, and research suggests that women with a history of sexual or physical violence are more likely to experience negative social and physical consequences following HIV-disclosure (Gielen et al., 2000). Other studies have documented associations between histories of partner violence and resistance to HIV-testing among women, even though the prospect of partner notification itself is not cited by these women as a barrier to testing (Maher et al., 2000). Internationally, studies suggest that less than a quarter of women who learn their status through perinatal testing disclose their status to their partners within the eighteen months following diagnosis (Maman, Mbwambo, Hogan, Kilonzo, & Sweat, 2001).

Current policy surrounding partner notification makes exceptions in contract tracing if potential violence is reported or suspected. However, this exception does not address the fact that the HIV-positive individual must then hide his/her status from an individual who is often her or his main partner. While contract tracing becomes impossible from the public health perspective, disclosure remains a critical issue for the newly diagnosed individual. Transforming partner notification programs into services that provide sustained support for disclosure over time would be much more beneficial. In addition, such sustained support in disclosure might help HIV-infected individuals develop strategies for informing new partners, as new relationships develop. Currently, research suggests that many HIV-infected individuals, especially younger people, delay disclosure to partners or family members until their disease has progressed significantly (O'Brien et al., 2003). A comprehensive disclosure-support program might help HIV-infected individuals weigh the relative risks of disclosure with the benefits of having those close to them aware of the demands they are facing in managing a chronic illness. By increasing the role of infected individuals in the partner notification process, behavioral interventions linked to partner notification have the potential to reduce transmission by affecting: (1) the infected index patient; (2) the notified partner; and (3) the discordant couple.

PARTNER NOTIFICATION REDEFINED: A RISK-REDUCTION PROGRAM

This acknowledgement of the future partners, and ongoing disclosure needs of HIV-infected individuals highlights the extent to which the locus of control over prevention efforts has shifted (c.f. Indyk & Golub, this volume). Behaviors that are thought of as disease management for HIV-infected individuals–adherence to drug treatment, safer needle use, safer sexual practices–double as prevention efforts for their uninfected partners by reducing the risk of HIV-transmission and of the transmission of drug-resistant viral strains. Guidelines from the Centers for Disease Control and Prevention recommend the incorporation of risk assessment and prevention counseling into the standard of care for HIV-infected individuals (CDC, 2003).

Similarly, partner notification services need to be redefined as part of an HIV-positive individual's risk-reduction plan. Studies demonstrate that partner notification, as it is currently utilized, has met with only limited public health success. A large scale analysis of partner notification data from 28 metropolitan areas revealed that health departments interview approximately 32% of individuals with newly reported HIV infection (Golden, Hogben, Potterat, & Handsfield, 2004). Ten-percent of the partners contacted as a result of these interviews tested HIV-positive, for an average of about 14 persons interviewed to identify one new case of HIV (Golden et al., 2004). However, the authors note that areas in which a large percentage of new cases are among men who have sex with men report the lowest rates of identification of new cases.

In addition, research suggests that partner notification services are least suited to dynamics which are contributing to recent increases in STI and HIV-infection rates. A review of the evidence available on the effectiveness of partner notification concludes that partner notification is a relatively ineffective means of disease control when sex with anonymous partners is common, when there is considerable delay before contacts can be traced, and when health services are inaccessible or unacceptable to clients (Cowan et al., 1996). Both CDC (1991) and state-specific studies (Andrus et al., 1990) have found limitations of the ability of partner notification strategies to reduce epidemics of other sexually transmitted diseases, such as syphilis.

In contrast, several studies have demonstrated that partner notification services that involve both partners in a discussion both of sero-status and of risk-reduction practices can significantly increase rates of condom use over time. In a longitudinal study examining the effects of partner notification on risk-reduction behavior and partnership dissolution, partner notification that involved both members of a couple was associated with higher condom use at six months, compared with couples in which only the HIV-positive partner received counseling services. In addition, these couples were less likely to break-up over the six month period of the study (Hoxworth, Spencer, Peterman, Craig, Johnson, & Maher, 2003).

In addition, partner notification services can be redefined to target risk-reduction. Studies have demonstrated that HIV-positive individuals are significantly less likely to disclose an HIV-diagnosis to a casual partner as compared to a main partner (O'Brien et al., 2003), and many patients report that they do not feel a moral responsibility to disclose a new diagnosis to past, casual partners (Cason et al., 2003). Given these realities, several cities are pioneering innovative methods of partner notification. In Los Angeles, the health department is attempting to use the Internet to identify anonymous partners using email. In a recent case report (CDC, 2004), between 29% (26/111) and 50% (7/13) of partners who received emails responded. In Seattle, a new program of HIV counseling and testing within bathhouses includes partner notification as part of its services (Spielberg, Branson, Goldbaum, Kurth, & Wood, 2003). Both these programs represent approaches to integrating partner notification with risk-reduction for contacts as well as index patients.

ETHICAL CONSIDERATIONS

As both the role of infected individuals and the time frame for partner notification efforts expand, advances in HIV diagnosis and treatment also have a series of implications on the ethics of partner notification. The argument over partner notification has largely been situated in the field of ethics and has centered on the responsibility of infected individuals to inform sexual and needle-sharing partners of their HIV status. In reexamining the partner notification process, both practical and moral considerations must be discussed.

For example, as viral load testing becomes routine, many individuals are being told that their viral load has been reduced to "undetectable levels." Research suggests that individuals with lower viral load are less infectious to others, since they have a lower concentration of virus in their blood stream and bodily fluids (Baeten & Overbaugh, 2003). While an individual with undetectable viral load may have an ethical responsibility to disclose his HIV status to past partners, does he have the same responsibility to disclose to current and future partners? While this article has not discussed the physician's role in the partner notification process, ethical analyses of partner notification write extensively about the physician's "duty to warn" (Gostin & Curan, 1987). Do physicians have the same responsibilities to notify the partners of their patients with low or high viral loads? A physician may decide that she has a stronger moral imperative to notify a patient's *past* partners (during a period when his viral load was high) than she does to notify the patient's *current* partner (who is still being exposed, but with undetectable levels of virus).

The complexity of drug treatment for HIV infection presents an added dimension to the concept of disclosure. What are the ethical responsibilities of individuals and physicians around disclosure of treatment failure? For example, let us assume that an individual has informed her partner that she is infected and the couple has decided to engage in intercourse, but always to use condoms. If the infected individual discovers that she is drug resistant, is she morally obligated to re-notify her partner? On the one hand, the fact that she is drug resistant changes the calculus of risk-taking; her partner is now risking infection with a virus that will not respond to therapy. On the other hand, she is still taking the same precautions to avoid transmission to her partner. By accepting the risk inherent in protected intercourse with an HIV positive individual, is the partner implicitly accepting additional risk? Or is the additional risk so great that knowledge cannot be waived? Physicians may be faced with the question of whether their moral responsibility to warn an uninfected partner extends to information regarding the emergence of drug resistance. Similar questions affect both infected individuals and their physicians as viral load fluctuates. There may a certain increase in viral load that warrants an additional notification.

As discussed above, HIV-infected individuals' commitment to risk reduction around sexual and needle use practices and adherence to drug treatment regimens can simultaneously fulfill treatment and prevention goals. Partner notification can be considered a third behavior which can similarly integrate these goals. However, there is a fundamental difference between partner notification and the other two behaviors; both risk reduction and adherence to treatment regimens directly benefit infected individuals by reducing the risk of disease progression. Partner notification, however, does not directly benefit HIV-positive individuals except to the extent that it is "the ethical thing to do" (Potterat, Meheus, & Gallwey, 1991). If infected individuals are to become true partners in prevention, the moral dilemmas inherent in the partner notification process must continue to challenge the creation of process, programs, and policy.

At the same time, discussions of the moral obligations inherent in partner notification and disclosure must be careful not to create situations that exacerbate the criminalization of sexual behavior by HIV-positive individuals. As of 2004, twenty states have passed legislation making it a crime for HIV-positive individuals to engage in sexual contact that presents a significant risk of HIV transmission, and fourteen states have made this behavior a felony (ACLU, 2004). Each of these laws has an exception for "informed consent," but the implications of this type of legislation are potentially dire. There is a danger that a realization of the critical role of HIV-infected individuals in prevention goals will place an undue burden without providing adequate supports for risk-reduction.

PARTNER NOTIFICATION AS PART OF THE CONTINUUM OF CARE

From a public health perspective, both *retrospective* and *prospective* partner notification is critical to HIV prevention efforts. Partner notification must be seen not only as a public health strategy for notifying those already exposed, but also as an opportunity for engaging and supporting infected HIV-positive individuals in the lifelong process of negotiating their lives in the context of their infection. Partner notification provides an invaluable opportunity to respond to the future of the epidemic; however, this response must include not only the creation of new programs to serve those infected and affected by the HIV epidemic, but a reexamination of the process through which services and supports are provided. A true expansion of the preventive case management model would involve targeted and sustained support for all *three* behaviors critical to the management of HIV: (1) adherence to medication regimens; (2) risk reduction around sexual behavior and needle use; and (3) retrospective and prospective partner notification and negotiation.

The incorporation of partner notification into the continuum of care exemplifies the integration of prevention and care for both HIV-positive and HIV-negative individuals. For infected individuals, this linkage integrates prevention into the care process; individuals engage in prevention/disclosure activities in the context of the care and management of their illness. For uninfected individuals (notified partners), the linkage integrates care into the process of prevention; individuals receive counseling and support in managing/maintaining their negative status, in addition to traditional risk reduction. A redefinition of the partner notification process would allow HIV-infected individuals to be better supported in their ongoing processes of both disclosure and risk-reduction.

REFERENCES

Andrus, J.K., Fleming, D.W., Harger, D.R., Chin, M.Y., Bennett, D.V., Honran, J.M., Oxman, G., Olson, B., & Foster, L.R. (1990). Partner Notification: Can It Control Epidemic Syphilis? *Annals of Internal Medicine, 7*, 539-543.

American Civil Liberties Union (2004). State criminal statutes on HIV transmission–2004. Author. Accessed on July 6, 2005, *http://www.aclu.org/HIVAIDS/HIVAIDS.cfm?ID=17769&c=21*

Bayer, R., & Toomey, K.E. (1992). HIV prevention and the two faces of partner notification. *American Journal of Public Health, 82*, 1158-1164.

Cason, C., Orrock, N., Schmitt, K., Tesoriero, J., Lazzarini, Z., & Sumartojo, E. (2002). The impact of laws on HIV and STD prevention. *The Journal of law, medicine & ethics: A journal of the American Society of Law, Medicine & Ethics, 30* (3 Suppl), 139-45.

Centers for Disease Control, Alternative Case-Finding Methods in a Crack-Related Syphilis Epidemic Philadelphia, 40 MMWR 5:77 (1991).

Centers for Disease Control and Prevention (2003). Incorporating HIV prevention into the medical care of persons living with HIV: recommendations of CDC, the Health Resources and Services Administration, the National Institutes of Health, and the HIV Medicine Association of the Infectious Diseases Society of America. *MMWR Morbidity and Mortality Weekly Report, 52* (RR-12), 1-24.

Cowan, F.M., French, R., & Johnson, A.M. (1996). The Role and Effectiveness of Partner Notification in STD Control: A Review. *Genitourinary Medicine, 72*(4), 247-52.

Dimas, J.T., & Richland, J.H. Partner notification and HIV infection: misconceptions and recommendations. *AIDS & Public Policy Journal.* 1989;4:206-217.

Gielen, A.C., Fogarty, L., O'Campo, P., Anderson, J., Keller, J., & Faden, R. (2000). Women living with HIV: disclosure, violence, and social support. *Journal of Urban Health, 77* (3), 480-491.

Golden, M.R., Hopkins, S.G., Morris, M., Holmes, K.K., & Handsfield, H.H. (2003). Support among persons infected with HIV for routine health department contact for HIV partner notification. *Journal of Acquired Immune Deficiency Syndromes, 32* (2), 196-202.

Golden, M.R., Hogben, M., Potterat, J.J., & Handsfield, H.H. (2004). HIV partner notification in the United States: A national survey of program coverage and outcomes. *Sexually Transmitted Diseases, 31* (12), 709-712.

Gostin L., & Curran, W.J. AIDS screening, confidentiality, and the duty to warn. *Am J Public Health.* 1987;77(3):361-65.

Hoxworth, T., Spencer, N.E., Peterman, T.A., Craig, T., Johnson, S., & Maher, J.E. (2003). Changes in partnerships and HIV risk behaviors after partner notification. *Sexually Transmitted Diseases, 30* (1), 83-88.

Indyk, D. & Golub, S.A. (2005). The Shifting Locus of Risk-Reduction: The Critical Role of HIV Infected Individuals. *Social Work in Health Care, 42*(3/4).

Landis, S.E., Schoenbach, V.J., Weber, D.J. et al. Results of a randomized trial of partner notification in cases of HIV infection in North Carolina. *NEJM.* 1992;326:101-106.

Maher, J.E., Peterson, J., Hastings, K., Dahlberg, L.L., Seals, B., Shelley, G., & Kamb, M.L. (2000). Partner violence, partner notification, and women's decisions to have an HIV test. *Journal of Acquired Immune Deficiency Syndromes, 25*(3), 276-282.

Maman, S., Mbwambo, J., Hogan, N.M., Kilonzo, G.P., & Sweat, M. (2001). Women's barriers to HIV-1 testing and disclosure: Challenges for HIV-1 voluntary counselling and testing. *AIDS Care, 13*(5), 595-603.

O'Brien, M.E., Richardson-Alston, G., Ayoub, M., Magnus, M., Peterman, T.A., & Kissinger, P. (2003). Prevalence and correlates of HIV serostatus disclosure. *Sexually Transmitted Diseases, 30*(9), 731-735.

Potterat, J.J., Meheus, A., & Gallwey, J. Partner notification: operational considerations. *Int J STD AIDS.* 1991; 2:411-415.

Ramstedt, K., Hallhagen, G., Ludin, B. et al. Contact tracing for Human Immunodeficiency Virus (HIV) infection. *STD.* 1990;17:37-41.

Spielberg, F., Branson, B.M., Goldbaum, G.M., Kurth, A. & Wood, R.W. (2003). Designing an HIV counseling and testing program for bathhouses: The Seattle experience with strategies to improve acceptability. *Journal of Homosexuality, 44* (3-4), 203-220.

The STARK Study:
A Cross-Sectional Study of Adherence
to Short-Term Drug Regimens
in Urban Kenya

Ann E. Ellis, BSE
Rebecca P. Gogel, AB
Benjamin R. Roman, BA
James B. Watson, MPH (candidate)
Debbie Indyk, PhD
Gary Rosenberg, PhD

SUMMARY. The purpose of the STARK study (Short-Term Adherence Research in Kenya) was to identify factors that predict adherence to short-term drug regimens in Nairobi, Kenya. The participants (N = 357) in the study were recruited from the RAFIKI Foundation Clinic, a free primary healthcare clinic in Kibera, Nairobi's largest slum. Quantitative surveys were administered to all the participants regarding their adherence patterns and to a subgroup of mothers (N = 233) regarding their adherence in giving medicine to their children. Forty participated in four

---

Ann E. Ellis, BSE, Rebecca P. Gogel, AB, Benjamin R. Roman, BA, James B. Watson, MPH (candidate), Debbie Indyk, PhD, and Gary Rosenberg, PhD, are affiliated with the Mount Sinai School of Medicine, New York, NY.

[Haworth co-indexing entry note]: "The STARK Study: A Cross-Sectional Study of Adherence to Short-Term Drug Regimens in Urban Kenya." Ellis, Ann E. et al. Co-published simultaneously in *Social Work in Health Care* (The Haworth Press, Inc.) Vol. 42, No. 3/4, 2006, pp. 237-250; and: *The Geometry of Care: Linking Resources, Research, and Community to Reduce Degrees of Separation Between HIV Treatment and Prevention* (ed: Debbie Indyk) The Haworth Press, Inc., 2006, pp. 237-250. Single or multiple copies of this article are available for a fee from The Haworth Document Delivery Service [1-800-HAWORTH, 9:00 a.m. - 5:00 p.m. (EST). E-mail address: docdelivery@haworthpress.com].

Available online at http://www.haworthpress.com/web/SWHC
© 2006 by The Haworth Press, Inc. All rights reserved.
doi:10.1300/J010v42n03_15

237

focus groups. Fifty-two percent of participants reported taking all of their prescribed medication and 47% took it until they felt better. Over 65% of mothers reported giving all prescribed medication to their children. The most frequently cited barriers to adherence included lack of food and clean water, stress, and financial problems. By identifying obstacles to adherence and strategies to overcome them, this study showed that a community-based clinic with committed healthcare workers in Kenya can empower an economically disadvantaged population to be adherent. *[Article copies available for a fee from The Haworth Document Delivery Service: 1-800-HAWORTH. E-mail address: <docdelivery@haworthpress.com> Website: <http://www.HaworthPress.com> © 2006 by The Haworth Press, Inc. All rights reserved.]*

KEYWORDS. Adherence, short-term medications, free clinic, Kibera, Kenya

BACKGROUND

In recent decades, increasing attention has been given to the methods and interventions that ensure successful delivery of medical care. In 2003, the World Health Organization issued a statement calling for action on improving adherence, described as "the extent to which a person's behavior–taking medication, following a diet, and/or executing lifestyle changes–corresponds with agreed recommendations from a health care provider" (WHO Report, 2003). The term "adherence" replaces its predecessor in the literature, "compliance," which was considered too punitive toward the patient. Since the therapeutic value of treatment cannot be optimized unless patients follow directions, low adherence results in both poor health outcomes and increased costs of health care.

The literature on adherence to medications for chronic diseases, such as HIV/AIDS and cancer, is extensive and presents several broad categories of "adherence predictors" that help to elucidate why some patients are adherent to medications while others are not. Some of these predictors include medication factors, psychological and social support factors, demographics and socioeconomic status and the nexus of culture, health, and illness. According to most published studies, on average 50% of patients worldwide adhere to the regimens (medicine, diet, exercise, etc.) prescribed by their health care provider, although more recent studies show an upward trend (WHO Report, 2003). Meta-analyses done prior to 1980 estimated the adherence rate in the United States to be roughly 63%; by 1998, it had risen to 76% (DiMatteo, 2004). The general consensus is that adherence is multi-factorial–involving the patient, the provider and the health care organization–and that adherence varies substantially by the particular condition and treatment.

Despite the extensive literature on medications for chronic diseases, there is a relative lack of research into short-term (less than two weeks) medication adherence. One critical study conducted in Ethiopia has already indicated that the problem of adherence extends to treatment plans regardless of their duration; in fact, it has been shown that adherence to short-term drugs deteriorates rapidly and that there is often a more immediate risk of overdose-related side effects and loss of efficacy among drugs taken for short-term courses (Abula, 2000). A select few other studies have examined adherence to antibiotics in disease-specific cases (Dunbar-Jacob, 2004; Cutler, 1984), but the scope of research into short-term adherence remains limited.

While the STARK study contributes to this knowledge base of short-term adherence patterns, what distinguishes it is its focus on the unique challenges to adherence in the setting of a free health clinic serving a disadvantaged urban population. A recent pilot study conducted at a public clinic in Brazil concluded that medical insufficiency continues to be an overwhelming problem in low-middle-income countries (Carmody et al., 2003), and Kenya is clearly no exception. However, another East African study conducted in the same year argued that in fact, the financial burden of purchasing medicine is not wholly, or even mostly, responsible for poor adherence rates (Salako et al., 2003). The STARK study elaborated a different hypothesis based not solely on resources, but instead on the idea that patients can be willing partners in adherence and illness prevention, and that the gap between having medicine and taking it faithfully may lie in the free clinic infrastructure. More important than actual adherence rates were the predictors of adherence and non-adherence as self-reported by participants; in other words, the reasons *why* some subjects were adherent and some were not. The interplay among culture and adherence is complex and dynamic, and thus the question of whether partnerships can be forged between clinic and patient was explored in tandem with specific adherence patterns.

RESEARCH PLAN

Participants and Setting

Participants were recruited from the RAFIKI Foundation Clinic, a primary health care facility that services residents of Kibera, the largest slum in Sub-Saharan Africa (population approximately one million). The clinic is supported by the RAFIKI Foundation, Inc., a non-profit foundation that became incorporated in 2001. In addition to the clinic, the Foundation also supports a free primary school and provides an avenue for students from the United States to serve at the school and clinic.

Every adult over 18 years old who came to the clinic during the dates of the study was invited to participate in the STARK study.

Methods

The research questions were addressed with two quantitative surveys. These were tested for clarity and timing using individuals not involved in this research project. One quantitative survey was designed to identify the factors that predict the adherence to short-term drug regimens for adults (N = 357) and a second survey was given to a subgroup of mothers (N = 233) regarding their adherence in giving medicine to their children. The quantitative surveys elicited information about the participants' demographics and socio-economic status, general attitudes toward health and health care workers, recent medical history and adherence patterns. The participants ranked the factors affecting their adherence to short-term drug regimens on a Likert scale. These surveys took on average 20-25 minutes to complete when administered together. A Kenyan nurse from the clinic explained the details of the study to potential participants, including the study objectives, compensation, informed consent process and administration. For every survey completed, the participants received a 500 g box of fortified porridge. In order to be as inclusive as possible, the study was designed so that participants had a choice of four methods for completing the quantitative surveys: They could read it themselves in Swahili or English, with a medical student present to answer any questions, or they could have it read to them in Swahili or English by a medical student. Four focus groups (N = 40) were also conducted to further probe the answers from the quantitative surveys. Medical students and doctors at the University of Nairobi Medical School translated all materials into Swahili.

Statistical Analysis

The randomized and anonymous data were analyzed using SPSS. Medians, means, and standard deviations were calculated for continuous variables. Univariate analysis was performed, including *t* tests for continuous factors, chi-square ratios, prevalence odds ratios (OR), and 95% confidence intervals (CI) for categorical factors. Logistic regression analysis was used to determine the prevalence odds ratios for univariate cofactors. All *p* values reported are two-tailed. A *p* value of < 0.05 was considered significant.

RESULTS

Study Population

The participants in this research belonged to Nairobi's lowest socio-economic class. In the adult study, 93% of participants were women and most of them came to the clinic with one or more of their children. 80% of adult participants were under the age of 30. 60% had attended upper primary school. The average weekly income was $2.50, and average weekly expenses were triple that amount. Seventy-seven percent of the participants received financial support from either a spouse or a family member. Other characteristics of the sample are described in Table 1.

The first aim of this study was to identify the specific barriers to adherence in this adult urban population:

The illnesses most frequently reported included malaria (64%), gastrointestinal illness (44%) and respiratory infections (34%). As depicted in Figure 1, the factors most frequently identified as barriers impeding adherence included: financial problems (74%), lack of food (58%), stress (48%), lack of clean water (42%) and transportation problems (44%).

Increasing education level was correlated with increasing perception that the following factors were barriers to adherence: living arrangements, job, stress, grieving and medication factors such as taste and size of pill (p < 0.05). Increasing age correlated with the increasing percep-

TABLE 1. Demographics of the 357 Participants of the STARK STUDY

Characteristic	n (%)
Females	331 (92.5)
18-30 years old	296 (80.1)
Married	286 (79.9)
Has one or more children	343 (96.4)
Post upper primary school education	95 (26.6)
Unemployed	215 (60.2%)
Weekly Income < 200 Ksh ($2.50)	222 (63.4%)

tion that key barriers to adherence were job concerns, financial problems and cost of medication (p < 0.05). The more control one feels over his or her health, the more positively he or she describes his or her overall health (p < 0.01).

The second aim of this study was to explore the specific barriers that impact a mother's ability to administer medication to her children:

The 233 women who enrolled in the mother/child aspect of the study were asked to answer questions in relation to either the child accompanying them or their oldest child. The average child's age was 4.1 years, 49% were male. The majority of the illnesses that they sought treatment for were malaria (63%), influenza (47%), respiratory infection (34%), stomach problems/diarrhea (55%) and skin problems (22%). Fifty percent of the children had been sick 1-3 times in the last six months, 42% had been sick more than three times. The two barriers to adherence identified by participants were: lack of nutritional food (52%) and trouble understanding instructions for medication use (41%).

Figure 2 illustrates the comparison of the barriers that impact a mother's ability to administer medication to her children compared with the mother's ability to take her own medication as prescribed.

The third aim of this study was to determine whether the barriers to adherence were the same for adults as for their children: .

The data from the mother/child surveys were compared to the adult surveys in order to elucidate differences between how mothers care for themselves versus their children. Fifty-nine percent of the mothers sought medical care for their child every time he or she was sick whereas only 35%

FIGURE 1. Key Barriers for Adults Taking Medicine

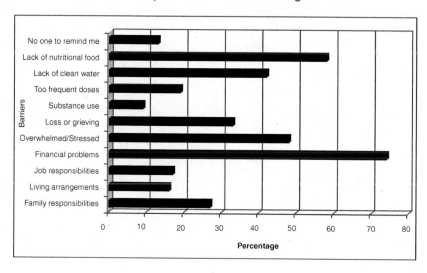

FIGURE 2. Key Barriers for Adults Taking Medication and Mothers Giving Their Children Medication

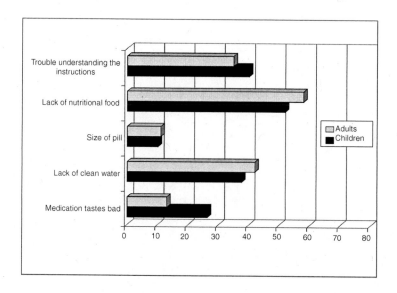

sought medical care for themselves when they were sick. Sixty-seven percent of the mothers gave all prescribed medication to their child whereas only 55% took all of their own medication. There is a positive relationship between overall perception of their own health and their perception of their child's health. Lack of food was a pervasive barrier to adherence for both groups.

> *The fourth aim of this study was to analyze whether a disadvantaged population in an urban slum could be adherent to short-term medication:*

The research showed that patients can, in fact, be adherent to an extent, but not to an extent that ensures optimal health. Given the recent concern about the development of antibiotic resistance among common acute pathogens, not fulfilling a full course of antibiotics may create even greater health hazards. Fifty-two percent of adults reported taking all of their prescribed medication and 47% took it until they felt better. Sixty-seven percent of mothers reported that their child takes all of his or her medication as prescribed.

As seen in Table 2, univariate analysis was used to determine factors affecting the level of achievable adherence in the study population.

DISCUSSION OF QUALITATIVE FINDINGS

Economically disadvantaged and resource-poor communities often have less access to health care and more constraints on their limited finances and social support. This observation may lead to the logical, but perhaps unfounded conclusion that people of a lower socio-economic status tend to be less adherent to medications prescribed to them. Why is it, then, that the patient population of the RAFIKI Foundation Clinic has statistical adherence rates in keeping with, and in some cases higher than, the general findings in the literature on adherence studies for patients who are largely of a higher socio-economic status? The findings from the STARK study suggest that there are distinct positive and negative predictors of adherence and that attitudes and behaviors about health and medicine also impact adherence patterns.

TABLE 2. Adherence to Short-Term Drug Regimens at the RAFIKI Foundation Clinic, Kenya, and Univariate Logistic Regression Analysis

Category	Takes All the Medicine as Prescribed	Takes Medication as Prescribed Until He/She Feels Better	OR (95% CI)[a]	p value[b]
Male	9	16	0.60 (0.26, 1.40)	0.23
Female	157	167	1.00	
Age 18-30	132	125	1.80 (1.11, 2.94)	0.02
Age > 30	34	58	1.00	
Married	143	137	2.09 (1.20, 3.63)	0.01
Not married	23	46	1.00	
No children	6	6	1.08 (0.34, 3.41)	0.90
One or more children	158	170	1.00	
Unemployed	94	117	0.74 (0.48, 1.13)	0.16
Employed	72	66	1.00	
Upper primary school and below	117	124	1.15 (0.71, 1.87)	0.60
Secondary school or higher	41	50	1.00	
Rarely boils water	74	71	1.27 (0.83, 1.94)	0.27
Usually boils water	92	112	1.00	
Not enough food	128	125	1.56 (0.97, 2.52)	0.07
Enough food	38	58	1.00	
Difficult to access health care	43	59	0.74 (0.46, 1.17)	0.20
Not difficult to access health care	122	123	1.00	
Comfortable with health care professionals	152	160	1.48 (0.62, 3.51)	0.38
Uncomfortable with health care professionals	9	14	1.00	
Understand doctor's instructions	151	151	2.31 (1.16, 4.60)	0.02
Do not understand doctor's instructions	13	30	1.00	
Believe it is very important to take medicine	160	180	0.44 (0.11, 1.81)	0.26
Do not believe it is very important to take medicine	6	3	1.00	
In poor or very poor health	74	58	1.39 (0.71, 2.73)	0.34
In good or excellent health	22	24	1.00	
Has control over his/her health	105	98	1.51 (0.98, 2.32)	0.06
Does not have control over his/her health	59	83	1.00	

[a] All odds ratios are univariate and should be interpreted as odds of taking all the medication as prescribed.
[b] p values for continuous variables are two-sided t tests for difference of means.

Positive Predictors

The RAFIKI Foundation Clinic employs a number of interventions and services that its patients unanimously agree lead to higher than expected adherence rates to short-term drug regimens. The services that make it easier for these patients to take their medicine as prescribed include the free fortified porridge, caring doctors, free medicine, good instructions and the counseling they receive from the nurse on how best to take the medicine. As one woman stated, "I have personally very much benefited from the porridge that they give out here. I feel better and have increased my strength and put on weight since I've been coming here and eating the porridge. This clinic has helped me to gain some control over my health." Another said, "The porridge gives me the necessary energy to be able to go home to take care of my children." A third woman—and a mother—recounted an experience that many of the other mothers had experienced: "My child who is almost four years old could not walk three months ago, and then once I started bringing her to this clinic to eat the fortified porridge, she quickly started getting healthier and gaining weight and feeling better. Now she can walk and even run!"

In addition, the study participants reported that having good dependable jobs would make it easier for them to take their medications on schedule because it would enable them to have enough good food and stability in their life. They feel that if they had good control over their finances, their health would be better.

Negative Predictors/Barriers

The greatest barrier to adherence cited by the adult study participants is a lack of food. For the majority of these women, it is a major problem that prevents them from taking their medication as prescribed. Lack of water, lack of money, stress, marital problems and forgetfulness also impede their ability to take their medication on time, though they try not to let these factors become major set-backs. Many of the subjects stated that they do not stop taking their medicine because of bad side-effects unless these side-effects are too severe. Pill size, bitter tasting medicine, pill burden and medicines that require bed rest, however, do make it harder for them to take their medication.

As expected, financial hardship is also a major barrier to adherence in this population. All of the women find it very difficult to support themselves. Most try to support themselves through small businesses: selling vegetables and fruit, washing clothes and plaiting hair. "Any money I get finishes so fast and there is so much to do," commented one woman. It is a big financial burden to come to the clinic, since they have to give up a whole day of work. The issue of losing work time is a top concern among mothers especially, whose daytime activities sometimes interfered with giving their children medication if the medication needed to be taken three times per day. Medication that has to be given to children during lunchtime was noted to be especially problematic. This finding supports a previous study conducted within the United States that showed that flexibility of clinic hours and shortened time between patient visits was found to be as important as the availability and simple dosing of medications (Falkenstein et al., 2004). Falkenstein et al. showed that poor adherence in children post-liver transplant was significantly reduced when clinics were open at more convenient hours for parents and when medical protocols were simplified.

Health Attitudes and Behaviors

The adults in this study firmly believe that western medicine plays a major role in their getting well. All the women agreed that taking medication is very important in order for them to get better. They feel it is very important to take the medications that they are given as prescribed and they usually take all of the medication that is given to them. When asked about the extent to which they feel they have control over their health, most of the women agreed that their financial instability diminishes their ability to have any control over their health. The women did state, however, that having doctors who are competent and caring, as they do at the RAFIKI Foundation Clinic, is instrumental in their feeling better about their health.

Health behaviors varied among the study participants. The amount of time and money the women have and the severity of the illness, determines whether or not they come to see a health care worker when they are sick. "I wait to see if I can weather out the illness. I only go to see a doctor if the situation worsens," stated one participant. Though they agreed that it is good to see a doctor for a regular, general check-up even if they are not sick, none of the women have ever come for a yearly check-up before due to lack of funds and some even find it absurd to ask the doctor for a check-up when they are not sick.

For those women who have any medication left over, some throw it out because they believe that the medicine would have expired by the time they would need it again, a few give any remaining medication to their neighbors and some keep it for themselves to use in the future. None of the women sell the remaining medication because they believe it is morally inappropriate. Mothers tend to be among the group that saves leftover medicine for future use: "What if my child falls ill at midnight?"

Mother/Child Findings

The data collected from the mother/child survey and focus groups tended to reinforce the data from the adult groups, with some interesting additions. As with the adult population, lack of food, financial resources, and time compromise the ability of mothers to adhere to a child's medication schedule. The mothers in this study believe medication is very important for their children to get well, and in fact, the mothers find it more important for their children to take their medicine than for themselves. "My child's health is paramount," exclaimed one mother. "If my child is sick, he needs to take the medication in order to get better, so even if the medicine has undesirable effects, I cannot stop giving my child the medicine." Most of the mothers believe that their children's health is better than their own health. "If I had only 20 Ksh. (equivalent to $0.25), I would spend it on medication for my child. I'd rather use my money for my child's health and see what becomes of my illness," remarked one mother. Most of the mothers feel they have more control over their child's health than they do over their own health.

Certain unique challenges were noted by the mothers. They reported that sometimes they just forget to give their children all their medication and many admit it is easier to take medicine themselves than it is to give it to their children. If the pill is large in size, or if the medicine has a bitter taste, the mothers said it could be exceedingly difficult to have their children take it. If the child refuses to take his or her medicine, some of the mothers force them or plead with the child to take the medication. Some of the children do have bad reactions to the medicine, so they stop taking the medicine and go back to see the doctor.

Despite the mothers concern for their child's welfare and their insistence that seeking health care for their children is a priority for them, most reported that they take their children to see a doctor only when the illness is very serious; this hesitation to seek medical care early may at least partially explain why so many children in Kibera do not receive the necessary medical care. Nevertheless, when seriously ill the mothers all believe in western medication to cure their children. The mothers said they would not take their children to a traditional healer because they believe "those people are just out for money and do not help to make my child well. Medicine that the doctor prescribes is what makes my child better." They feel very comfortable bringing their children to see the doctor at the RAFIKI Foundation clinic and they feel more comfortable bringing their children to see the doctor than they feel going to see the doctor themselves. They confide in their doctor about their children's medical health, but not about their children's personal problems.

CONCLUSION

This study investigated whether partnerships can be developed with patients to improve adherence in a free clinic setting. It explored the feasibility of conducting adherence research at free clinics and sought input from participants through focus groups. The investigators were welcomed by an enthusiastic group of patients at the RAFIKI Foundation Clinic who were eager to participate in the research study, both by filling out questionnaires and by participating in focus groups. More people wanted to participate than time and resources permitted. The study outcome shows that clinics that are responsive to their populations are, indeed, able to form strong partnerships with their patients. The RAFIKI Foundation Clinic has established enormous trust between its patients and its doctors and staff, which has facilitated the provision of health care and the implementation of this study. Furthermore, this model of a locally staffed, externally funded clinic may succeed in avoiding an important problem raised in a recent JAMA article, which pointed out that aid to resource-poor nations needs to be delivered in a sustainable form in accord with the local level of care (Kent et al., 2004). The authors of that paper posited that HIV studies in Africa, while scientifically relevant, are unrealistic if the sample population is unable to access or sustain treatment with the same drugs at the end of the clinical trial period. It is the intent of the researchers involved in the STARK study that the findings will directly impact the patients at the RAFIKI Foundation Clinic, leading to better adherence and ultimately, better health outcomes.

There are limitations in the present work, specifically related to the fact that the research was conducted among a primarily non-English speaking population. Although all the study instruments were carefully translated into Swahili, it is possible that some information on the questionnaires was not adequately conveyed from translator to participant. The potential for such misunderstanding may have been alleviated, at least in part, by testing the questionnaires on the Kibera population rather than on an independent, non-Swahili-speaking group.

The findings of this exploratory study should lead to further research in adherence to short-term medication addressing the following questions: Is adherence impacted by the patient/provider relationship? Do patients demonstrate greater adherence to medications that are prescribed by someone they know and trust? How can the lessons learned about short-term adherence be used to improve long-term adherence?

The findings from the STARK study provide strong evidence that there are specific yet surmountable barriers to adherence that can be targeted for intervention and that a disadvantaged population can be motivated to improve adherence patterns when given the support of a committed, community-based clinic.

REFERENCES

Abula, T. (2000). Patient noncompliance with therapeutic regimens and the factors of noncompliance in Gondar. Gondar, Ethiopia. *Ethiopian Journal of Health Development, 14*(1), 1-6.

Carmody, E.R, Diaz, T., Starling, P., dos Santos, A.P., & Sacks, H.S. (2003). An evaluation of antiretroviral HIV/AIDS treatment in a Rio de Janeiro public clinic. *Tropical Medicine and International Health, 8*(5), 378-385.

Cutler, A.F. & Schubert, T.T. (1993). Patient factors affecting Helicobacter pylori eradication with triple therapy. *American Journal of Gastroenterology, 88*(4), 505-509.

DiMatteo, M.R. (2004). Variations in patients' adherence to medical recommendations: A qualitative review of 50 years of research. *Medical Care, 42*(3).

Dunbar-Jacob, J., Sereika, S.M., Foley, S.M., Bass, D.C., & Ness, R.B. (2004). Adherence to oral therapies in pelvic inflammatory disease. *Journal of Womens Health, 13*(3), 285-91.

Falkenstein, K., Flynn, L., Kirkpatrick, B., Casa-Melley, A., & Dunn, S. (2004). Noncompliance in children post-liver transplant. Who are the culprits? *Pediatric Transplant, 8*(3), 233-236.

Kent, D.M., Mwamburi, M., Bennish, M.L., Kupelnick, B., & Ioannidids, J.P.A. (2004). Clinical trials in sub-saharan Africa and established standards of care: A systematic review of HIV, tuberculosis, and malaria trials. *Journal of the American Medical Association, 292*, 237-242.

Salako, B.L., Ajose, F.A., & Lawani, E. (2003). Blood pressure control in a population where antihypertensives are given free. *East African Medical Journal, 80*(10), 529-531.

WHO Report (2003). Adherence to Long-term Therapies: Evidence for Action. http://www.who.int/chronic_conditions/en/adherence_report.pdf

Index

BOOK ORDER FORM!

Order a copy of this book with this form or online at:
http://www.HaworthPress.com/store/product.asp?sku= 5796

The Geometry of Care
*Linking Resources, Research, and Community to Reduce Degrees
of Separation Between HIV Treatment and Prevention*

____ in softbound at $19.95 ISBN-13: 978-0-7890-3212-6 / ISBN-10: 0-7890-3212-0.

____ in hardbound at $34.95 ISBN-13: 978-0-7890-3211-9 / ISBN-10: 0-7890-3211-2.

COST OF BOOKS ____

POSTAGE & HANDLING ____
US: $4.00 for first book & $1.50
for each additional book
Outside US: $5.00 for first book
& $2.00 for each additional book.

SUBTOTAL ____

In Canada: add 7% GST. ____

STATE TAX ____
CA, IL, IN, MN, NJ, NY, OH, PA & SD residents
please add appropriate local sales tax.

FINAL TOTAL ____

If paying in Canadian funds, convert
using the current exchange rate,
UNESCO coupons welcome.

❑ BILL ME LATER:
Bill-me option is good on US/Canada/
Mexico orders only; not good to jobbers,
wholesalers, or subscription agencies.

❑ Signature ____

❑ Payment Enclosed: $____

❑ PLEASE CHARGE TO MY CREDIT CARD:

❑ Visa ❑ MasterCard ❑ AmEx ❑ Discover
❑ Diner's Club ❑ Eurocard ❑ JCB

Account # ____

Exp Date ____

Signature ____
(Prices in US dollars and subject to change without notice.)

PLEASE PRINT ALL INFORMATION OR ATTACH YOUR BUSINESS CARD

Name	
Address	
City	State/Province ____ Zip/Postal Code
Country	
Tel	Fax

May we use your e-mail address for confirmations and other types of information? ❑Yes ❑No We appreciate receiving
your e-mail address. Haworth would like to e-mail special discount offers to you, as a preferred customer.
We will never share, rent, or exchange your e-mail address. We regard such actions as an invasion of your privacy.

Order from your **local bookstore** or directly from
The Haworth Press, Inc. 10 Alice Street, Binghamton, New York 13904-1580 • USA
Call our toll-free number (1-800-429-6784) / Outside US/Canada: (607) 722-5857
Fax: 1-800-895-0582 / Outside US/Canada: (607) 771-0012
E-mail your order to us: orders@HaworthPress.com

For orders outside US and Canada, you may wish to order through your local
sales representative, distributor, or bookseller.
For information, see http://HaworthPress.com/distributors

(Discounts are available for individual orders in US and Canada only, not booksellers/distributors.)

Please photocopy this form for your personal use.
www.HaworthPress.com

BOF06